40.98

REFLECTIONS ON
PALLIATIVE CARE

Oct 22

Series editor: David Clark, Professor of Medical Sociology,
University of Sheffield

The subject of death in late modern culture has become a rich field of
theoretical, clinical and policy interest. Widely regarded as a taboo until
recent times, death now engages a growing interest among social scientists,
practitioners and those responsible for the organization and delivery of
human services. Indeed, how we die has become a powerful commentary
on how we live and the specialized care of dying people holds an important
place within modern health and social care.

This series captures such developments in a collection of volumes which
has much to say about death, dying, end-of-life care and bereavement in
contemporary society. Among the contributors are leading experts in death
studies, from sociology, anthropology, social psychology, ethics, nursing,
medicine and pastoral care. A particular feature of the series is its attention
to the developing field of palliative care, viewed from the perspectives of
practitioners, planners and policy analysts; here several authors adopt a multidisciplinary approach, drawing on recent research, policy and organizational
commentary, and reviews of evidence-based practice. Written in a clear,
accessible style, the entire series will be essential reading for students of
death, dying and bereavement and for anyone with an involvement in
palliative care research, service delivery or policy making.

Current and forthcoming titles:

David Clark, Jo Hockley, Sam Ahmedzai (eds): *New Themes in Palliative
Care*
David Clark and Jane Seymour: *Reflections on Palliative Care*
Mark Cobb: *Spiritual Issues in Palliative Care*
Kirsten Costain Schou and Jenny Hewison: *Experiencing Cancer: Quality
of Life in Treatment*
David Field, David Clark, Jessica Corner and Carol Davis (eds): *Researching
Palliative Care*
David Kissane and Sidney Bloch: *Family Grief Therapy*
Gordon Riches and Pamela Dawson: *An Intimate Loneliness: Supporting
Bereaved Parents and Siblings*
Tony Walter: *On Bereavement*

REFLECTIONS ON PALLIATIVE CARE

DAVID CLARK
JANE SEYMOUR

OPEN UNIVERSITY PRESS
Buckingham · Philadelphia

for
Diane and Jerry

Open University Press
Celtic Court
22 Ballmoor
Buckingham
MK18 1XW

email: enquiries@openup.co.uk
World wide web: http://www.openup.co.uk

and
325 Chestnut Street
Philadelphia, PA 19106, USA

First Published 1999

A catalogue record of this book is available from the British Library

ISBN 0 335 19454 0 (pbk)   0 335 19455 9 (hbk)

Library of Congress Cataloging-in-Publication Data

Clark, David, 1953–
    Reflections on palliative care : sociological and policy
perspectives / David Clark and Jane Seymour.
        p.   cm. — (Facing death)
    Includes bibliographical references and index.
    ISBN 0-335-19455-9 (hb). — ISBN 0-335-19454-0 (pbk)
    1. Palliative treatment—Sociological aspects.   2. Palliative
treatment—Political aspects.   3. Terminal care—Sociological
aspects.   4. Terminal care—Political aspects.   I. Seymour, Jane,
1958– . II. Title. III. Series.
    R726.8.C544   1999   98–28627 CIP
    362.1'75—dc21

Typeset by Graphicraft Limited, Hong Kong
Printed in Great Britain by Biddles Limited, Guildford and Kings Lynn

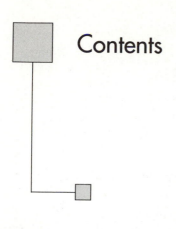

Contents

Series editor's preface   vii
Notes on the authors   ix
Acknowledgements   x

Introduction   1

Part I   Death in society   3
Introduction to Part I   5

1   The social meaning of death and suffering   8
    The world of experience   10
    Identity and the body   15
    Representations of suffering   17
    Dying in late modern culture   21
2   Ageing, dying and grieving   24
    Ageing and dying   25
    Informal care   32
    Bereavement, grief and mourning   40
3   The ethics of dying   47
    Euthanasia: historical and social perspectives   49
    Euthanasia: requests and responses   52

Part II   The philosophy and practice of palliative care   59
Introduction to Part II   61

4   History and development   65
    Late nineteenth- and early twentieth-century hospices   67

  A movement originates 69
  Global spread and redefinition 73
5 Definitions, components, meanings 79
  What is palliative care? 80
  The 'good death' 88
  The limits to palliation? 94
6 Routinization and medicalization 104
  The 'routinization' thesis 104
  The medicalization thesis 113
  Reappraising routinization and medicalization 118

Part III   Policy issues 125
Introduction to Part III 127

7 Policy development and palliative care 131
  The NHS and the early hospices 133
  Managing the NHS and managing terminal care 136
  An uneasy alliance 138
  The Conservative reforms and palliative care 140
  Some key issues in the 1990s 146
8 The delivery of palliative care services 151
  Hospital-based palliative care 152
  Palliative care at home 157
  In-patient hospices 165
  Institutional homes for older people 168

Part IV   Conclusions 173
Introduction to Part IV 175

9 The future for palliative care 176
  Some propositions about the future for palliative care 178
  Policy influences on future developments 181
  Unfinished agendas 185

References 188
Index 211

Series editor's preface

There can be no doubt that the hospice and palliative care movement represents one of the most important contributions to our thinking about death, dying and bereavement in the latter part of the twentieth century. The Facing Death series began with an overview of the current state of palliative care around the world in which Clark, Hockley and Ahmedzai (1997) drew together the writings of a diverse range of practitioners, planners and academic commentators. The second book in the series *Experiencing Cancer*, by Costain Schou and Hewison (1999) moved us away from concepts, models and theories and was firmly centred on the experiences of patients and their companions, as lived rather than as prescribed. In *Reflections on Palliative Care* David Clark and Jane Seymour seek to further extend our understanding of this rapidly expanding specialty and the ways in which it is affecting those it seeks to serve.

This book is written from the combined and overlapping perspectives of sociology and social policy and seeks to understand palliative care in two ways. First, it examines palliative care within the changing context of meanings, values and structures which make up what the authors refer to as *the dispositions of late modernity*. In this sense the book regards palliative care not only as a topic, but also as a resource for sociological enquiry. Commonly viewed as the solution to modern problems of death and terminal care, palliative care is also seen here as part of the wider sociological tensions surrounding our relationship to the question of human mortality in modern culture. Second the book shows how, despite its origins in a voluntary and independent hospice movement, palliative care has very quickly become caught up in the complex policy environment which surrounds it. This has called for adaptiveness in responding to successive waves of 'reform' to the health and social care system, common in the UK as in other affluent countries. Underpinning these sociological and policy perspectives, the authors also adopt a strongly historical frame of reference for their analysis. We are thus furnished with a detailed account of modern hospice and palliative care origins, which is central to their discussion of the philosophy and practice of palliative care and aids understanding of the rapid diversification which has taken place in the delivery of palliative care services.

Reflections on Palliative Care is a book by two authors clearly committed to the further development of the specialty they describe. Yet this commitment does not inhibit a critical and probing orientation. The book should therefore be of value to those seeking to go beyond the rhetoric which surrounds hospice and palliative care and who seek a more detailed and sustained analysis of past development and current dilemmas. In the final chapter, in particular, some propositions are developed about the future development of palliative care which may well provoke further discussion on the part of those involved. This book is clearly not the last word on the relationship between hospices, palliative care and the wider society. Rather it should be seen as the further extension of a debate which subsequent contributions to the Facing Death series will no doubt extend and elaborate.

David Clark

Notes on the authors

David Clark has wide-ranging interests in sociological aspects of religion, family life, health, illness and ageing. His current research and writing focuses on the history, development and impact of hospice and palliative care. He was appointed Professor of Sociology at Sheffield Hallam University in 1993 and then to the Chair of Medical Sociology in the Palliative Medicine Department of the University of Sheffield in 1995. He is the author and editor of numerous books and edits the *Facing Death* series for Open University Press.

Jane Seymour is a research associate in the Palliative Medicine Department of the University of Sheffield. She trained as a nurse in 1979, having completed a degree in Social Science at Exeter University. During her nursing career she worked mainly in acute care and intensive care: it was here that she developed an interest in end-of-life care, death, dying and bereavement. She gained a master's degree in sociology from Sheffield Hallam University, and in 1997 a doctorate from the University of Sheffield.

Acknowledgements

A variety of colleagues, friends and kin have supported our endeavours in writing this book and we owe them our thanks. Students on the Diploma/ MMedSci in Palliative Care at the University of Sheffield have helped us explore many of the issues we have covered here, and we are grateful to them for their enthusiasm and critical commentary. In recent years there has developed a growing community of interest in matters of death, dying and palliative care and fellow-travellers at many meetings and conferences have stimulated our thinking, for which we continue to be thankful. Closer to home we are fortunate indeed to have colleagues in the Sheffield Palliative Care Studies Group who come to their subject matter from several disciplinary perspectives within health care, the social sciences and the humanities; these together with others across the University of Sheffield have been of immeasurable support to the development of our ideas and thinking, in some cases over several years. Every day we each work closely with Margaret Jane, a secretarial colleague of immeasurable skill, patience and dedication; we thank Margaret not only for all her hard work on this book, but for everything else she contributes to the department and to our quality of life. Lastly, the book is dedicated to two very special people, who have heard it all before.

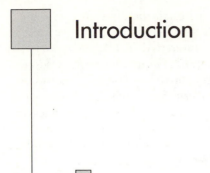

Introduction

This is a book written first and foremost for students of palliative care. We hope it will also interest practitioners, policy makers and researchers interested in the subject. It is a book of reflections and observations which draws on the perspectives of sociology and of health and social policy, and which in places adopts a markedly historical frame of reference. We are conscious that it is a contribution to a growing palliative care literature, and we hope it will add something new to the debate.

Our book has four parts, each of which has a summary introduction which readers may find helpful. In Part I, we consider dying and death as social phenomena deeply embedded within society as a whole. We have not attempted here a full sociological appraisal of the subject, rather we choose to focus on some key aspects of contemporary dying, exploring questions of ageing, informal care and bereavement as well as end-of-life care ethics. In Part II we attempt a detailed deconstruction of the philosophy and practice of palliative care, beginning with its historical development, considering questions of definition and examining some of the emergent pressures on this new specialty. In Part III our analysis shifts to broader questions of policy which are impacting upon palliative care and we examine the range of settings in which it is being delivered. In the final part of the book we seek to bring together our reflections around a single issue: the future for palliative care.

Since the formation of the first modern hospices in the late 1960s and early 1970s huge developments in the care of dying people and those close to them have been occurring. The rise of palliative care represents an attempt to adopt a multidimensional approach to care in the face of mortal illness, which takes into account physical, social, psychological and spiritual elements. We regard palliative care as closely intertwined with its culture and context. Our discussion in this book therefore focuses a great deal on the relationships between death and dying and palliative care *in the modern context*. Specifically we are interested in *late modernity*: we regard this as that fascinating border country between a *modern* world-view based on unproblematic notions of social progress, scientific ascendancy and 'the grand narrative', and the *post-modern* vista in which images, representations and discourse hold sway. *Late modernity* for us provides the context for reflecting upon and making sense of palliative care and we view the dispositions of late modern culture as essential to understanding whence palliative care has come and where it might be going.

This is not a book based on our own empirical studies, though we do refer to these on occasion. Nor does it deal with every aspect of palliative care. It does however attempt a detailed examination of adult palliative care from a sociological perspective, and we trust there will be some value in that.

David Clark and Jane Seymour

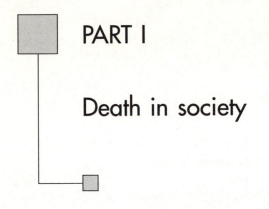

PART I

Death in society

Introduction to Part I

Our book opens with an appraisal of certain key themes within the contemporary sociological understanding of death and dying. We have not sought here a fully comprehensive overview of the subject, rather we have deliberately highlighted topics which relate to the broader purpose of the book, so we emphasize areas which seem particularly relevant to a full understanding of the development of palliative care to date, together with an assessment of its future prospects. In Part I therefore readers should give attention to the following four issues:

- The reflexive character of late modern identity and its implications for the social construction of illness, suffering and death.
- The importance of human ageing as a central characteristic allied to the experience of death and dying in late modern society.
- The creation of new patterns of dependency within society and within families and households.
- The emergence of an ethical debate on end-of-life care and the place of euthanasia.

These four themes, we believe, are highly relevant to the social context which is shaping the emerging theory and practice of palliative care, together with the surrounding policy context.

The starting point for our book is the claim that the understanding of death cannot be reduced to its biological parameters. Rather death, and particularly the process of dying, are located on the interface between biology and culture. So much so that many anthropologists and sociologists have seen death as the central binding agent within the fragile tissue of human society. It is awareness of our own mortality which somehow provides the preconditions for all human thought and action. In this sense death is not so much something that threatens society as something which makes society possible.

Partly for these reasons, the sociology of death has been the subject of renewed scholarly interest in recent years. Central to current discussions is a recognition of the importance of late modern culture for contemporary 'deathways'. In one sense, of course, death is a great universal, but there are huge variations in how it is manifested in traditional, modern and late (or post-) modern society. Several commentators are agreed that death poses particular kinds of problems for late modern identities. In Part I of the book we have chosen to approach this problem through a wider discussion of human suffering. This is a topic often ignored by sociologists, but its essentially social character is something which commends it to us. Suffering and death are of course not always combined, but for many they are uniquely conjoined. We suggest here that there is the potential to develop a moral order of suffering, in which late modern illness narratives play an important part.

The essential condition of late modern dying is that it is often protracted and comes at the end of a long life. Accordingly, the *trajectory* of dying becomes important and within it we see the valorization of certain key features – awareness, self-determination, reflexive heroism. One paradox of such a trajectory is that the grieving which can accompany death is brought forward and may manifest itself before the person has died by any biomedical definition. As we point out, however, such a trajectory may be more readily achieved in the context of death from a malignant disease and there are senses in which those whose lives are ended by other more protracted and more erratic conditions may constitute *the disadvantaged dying*.

Given the close interconnections between ageing and dying we are surprised at the lack of collaboration and exchange between professional students of these phenomena. Gerontologists and thanatologists rarely seem to meet up. Yet understanding dying has to involve understanding ageing and here we highlight three particular areas of importance. First, the political economy of old age encompasses questions of how older people relate to the labour market, to taxation and welfare systems and the ways in which discrimination occurs on grounds of age. Second, there is a need better to understand the life worlds of older people and to enhance appreciation of everyday experience, meanings, values, health and social care aspirations. Third, we highlight some of the important demographic trends (with associated misconceptions) that are influencing the place of older people within society.

The dying trajectory for many also incorporates the experience of significant others. For this reason we have included a discussion of the part which so-called 'informal carers' may play in the care of people who are dying. Many studies in recent years have showed how informal carers and the care they provide cannot be taken for granted. By *deconstructing* caring these commentators have shown how care relates to the division of labour within families and households and in particular how it forms part of the set of expectations associated with being a female relative. The close relationship between 'community care', 'family care' and 'care by women' is central to this.

Of course it is often 'informal carers' who bear the mantle of grief after a death has occurred, and yet this may coincide with the precise moment when health and social services and other social networks go into retreat, leaving the bereaved carer isolated and alone. We have tried here to distinguish the formal characteristics of bereavement (being deprived of someone) from grief (the emotional reactions which may ensue) and mourning (the socially sanctioned behaviours which accompany bereavement). There is no doubt the psychology and sociology of bereavement are currently moving through interesting times. The dominant bereavement paradigm of the twentieth century is based on processes of social and psychological restitution following an essential separation from the dead person. This is now being challenged in favour of models which give far greater emphasis to the bereaved person's continuing relationship with the deceased, and the continuing importance of the deceased in shaping the identities of those who live on.

Reflexivity in the dying process provides wider opportunities for a discussion of end-of-life care ethics. This is a fast-moving field, so we have tried to focus here on some broad underlying issues, rather than, for example, current aspects of legislation in any given context. Much of the discussion here revolves around the bigger question of whether, in what circumstances and by whom life can be ended deliberately. Various paradoxes appear. On the available evidence the public seem in favour of some forms of euthanasia. Certainly doctors and nurses are asked on occasions to administer it; and sometimes they do. Yet law makers remain nervous of change and where the law has been altered to a more liberal stance on euthanasia it has been quickly subject to counter-challenges. For a long time leaders of the hospice movement have argued that an extension of hospice practice would eliminate the demand for euthanasia. However, in the context of late modern trajectories of dying with their emphasis upon autonomy, and supported by a limited amount of empirical research evidence, this seems unlikely. Indeed, greater exposure to hospice care may make discussion of euthanasia more, rather than less, likely.

Part I of the book sets the scene for our subsequent exploration of palliative care in policy and practice. We try to get to grips with some aspects of late modern dying, from a sociological perspective. We hope to show that how we die is an extension of how we live and that in this particular framework any analysis must be alive to questions of reflexivity, of identity, of human ageing, of demographic transitions, and of ethical dilemmas at the end of life.

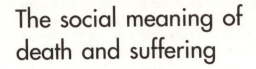

1 The social meaning of death and suffering

In the modern Western world many of us, at least until we undergo our own demise, will only ever have a limited experience of death. In the main we will encounter it indirectly, as if through a prism or filter. Consumed with the business of life, death hovers in our peripheral vision or confronts us at a tangent. So it is that death has little or no place in the day-to-day affairs of many, save for those experts who are trained and paid to deal with it, and who must somehow seek to manage its consequences. In this respect modern Westerners differ dramatically from both their predecessors in earlier times and their contemporaries elsewhere in the world. For the history of Western societies is littered with epidemics, war and natural disasters, just as these phenomena continue to beset the poorer countries of the world today. Paradoxically, in the West death has become largely *absent* from day-to-day experience and yet also *omnipresent*, in the mass media of newspapers, television, radio and film. In modern life the private and public dimensions of death therefore *appear* radically separated and this has wide-ranging consequences for how we respond to death and dying, both individually and collectively.

The sociologist Peter Berger once noted that 'every human order is a community in the face of death' (1973: 87). This observation contains a fundamental truth, but beyond it lie many paradoxes and subtleties. Human orders change in time and space; perceptions and experiences of 'community' are multifaceted; and even death itself can no longer be taken as a 'given' of biological existence, but has rather become a disputed territory where differing definitions and meanings are brought to bear. It is this very pluralization and fragmentation of aspects of death which makes it such an important subject for sociology and which may explain why, after years of relative neglect, we now seem to be moving into a period of new sociological interest in death studies.

Some writers have made the important point that, to be of any real worth, sociological thinking on death should be located within the broad concerns of the discipline as a whole, rather than confined inside a narrow sub-specialty. Thus Mellor argues that 'the task we must set ourselves in the sociology of death should be nothing less than that of contributing to the developing reassessments of, and debates surrounding, the strategies of sociology' (Mellor 1993: 12). More succinctly, Walter poses the question 'a sociology of death, or a mortal sociology?' (Walter 1993: 290).

There is undoubtedly a case for enriching wider sociological debates with a deeper awareness and understanding of human mortality. The sheer inevitability of death makes it a phenomenon of central importance to social scientists. By retaining this wider perspective we create opportunities to highlight ways in which dying, death and bereavement are socially constructed in relation to particular cultural, structural and historical circumstances. This perspective reminds us that the unique circumstances of an individual's death contain important external reference points. A recent collection of essays shows how these relate to well-known social indicators, such as gender, age, ethnicity, social class (Field *et al.* 1997). Other factors shaping the social experience of death involve aspects of the local community, available help and support, and the organization of formal health care systems. Beyond these lie wider belief systems, attitudes to death and the complex, shifting tapestry of meanings, values and representations of death in modern society. On this basis the interleaving of issues of mortality within the wider concerns of sociology makes a good deal of sense. Our understanding of family life, for example, is considerably impoverished if we ignore ways in which families respond to and deal with dying, death and bereavement. Similarly taking account of death and loss may enhance our understanding of particular social organizations – schools, factories, hospitals. Most obviously, the place of death within the analysis of global geo-political change is of central importance when addressing questions of war, genocide, oppression, 'ethnic cleansing' and famine. Such examples all support the notion of a sociology which is more death-conscious and more willing to integrate questions of mortality into the central area of its concerns.

At the same time, sub-specialization is a tendency which is difficult to resist. Almost inevitably, sociologists with a special interest in death are likely to gravitate together, and in developing their interests, to run the risk of isolation from more mainstream disciplinary concerns. This must be guarded against; but specialization also fosters benefits. Recent work has drawn attention to large areas about which detailed understanding from a sociological perspective is still in its infancy. Several of these will be dealt with in this book, particularly in Parts II and III, where we explore one particularly modern response to death in the form of the palliative care movement, with its specific set of underlying principles and systems of service organization. Sociological and policy interest in these areas has been relatively underdeveloped until the last few years, but now there are signs of a 'critical mass' of interested scholars whose activities are seen in publications, specialist meetings and the development of networks of individuals.

Perhaps then a 'mortal sociology' and a 'sociology of death' are both desirable. Certainly, the contents of our initial chapters will draw on both dimensions, hopefully in ways which benefit from the slightly different focus which each has to offer.

The world of experience

In either of these veins, there is a problem for sociology in focusing upon the *experience* of death, although it is easy to argue that this is the essential component from which a sociological analysis should proceed. We are thinking here of the circumstances in which death occurs: the responses made by individuals, households and wider social networks; the characteristic problems and practical difficulties which occur in facing death; as well as the existential dilemmas which it poses. Of course it quickly becomes apparent when considering these issues that experiences of death in complex modern societies are enormously varied and that it is far from easy to generalize about the ways in which individuals die and the social factors which have an influence. Indeed huge variation in the circumstances of death may be taken as one marker of what is itself termed 'modernity'. Giddens (1991) has pointed out that in what he calls 'late modernity' (the period in which we are living now) social arrangements are characterized by their dynamism, the degree to which they undercut traditional ways of thinking and acting, and their global ramifications. At the same time modernity has also altered the nature of everyday life and our own personal experiences. As Giddens puts it: 'One of the distinctive features of modernity, in fact, is an increasing inter-connection between the two "extremes" . . . globalising influences on the one hand and personal dispositions on the other' (1991: 1). In such a context, the manner in which we die takes on many possibilities: modernity offers a range of deathly scenarios.

Two extremes help to illustrate this point. On the one hand death in modern societies characterized by ageing populations may appear as a slow, wasting process which comes at the end of a long life. The gradual decline of an elderly person over a period of years, perhaps accompanied by a chronic illness leading to infirmity and high levels of dependence on others, is certainly a common image. In this sense we perhaps consider death as the final destination in a long journey. On the other hand modernity offers us innumerable examples of the journey cut short and of attenuated life. Of course, early death in pre-modern times was a commonplace, when infectious diseases and harsh social conditions combined to suppress life expectancy. Modernity's spectre however is of sudden death and is differently constructed, arising out of war, famine (often coupled with war), genocide and disaster. Mass death is frequently a component of this – hauntingly present in recent times on the killing fields of Rwanda and Bosnia. Sudden death on such a scale makes glaringly apparent the role of human agency and the influence of structural factors in determining patterns and dimensions of human mortality.

Between these two extremes of *gradual* and *catastrophic* death lies a third category, what we might call *premature* death. Included here are the 'everyday disasters' of modern life – road traffic and other accidental deaths, but also death from the diseases of modernity – HIV/AIDS, heart attack, cancer.

For descriptive purposes, we may seek to construct such 'categories' in order to see better the ways in which death manifests itself in the modern world. It is however a characteristic of our times that such distinctions and comparisons are frequently blurred in the world of experience. One aspect of the globalization of modern life has been to create informational links across widely dispersed groups of people. So it might be that the elderly Westerner, slowly dying at home, is confronted on the television news by the horrors of war on the other side of the world. Similarly television documentaries on cancer, AIDS and other health issues contribute to wider discourses of death and dying which in turn shape the experience of those affected personally by these diseases. In this way we see an interweaving between what C. Wright Mills referred to as 'private troubles and public issues' (1967). We see that our own individual, uniquely encountered pain and suffering, the beliefs we attribute to these and the life strategies adopted in response are also embedded in a wider context that goes well beyond our personal experience. Such complexities highlight the dangers of categorizing uncritically individuals as 'clients', 'patients', or 'informal carers' – labels which imply a mono-dimensional perspective which is capable of seeing human beings only in relation to the formal organizations of health and social care. Yet such reductionism may be the only way in which complex bureaucracies can continue to function in a context where so many aspects of modern culture appear as a speeding juggernaut, perilously out of control (Giddens 1990). In a 'runaway world' (Leach 1967) the manner of our dying may likewise depart from earlier pathways, careering madly into new and uncharted territory.

This book will be dealing with the implications of two of these three scenarios: gradual death and premature death. These seem to us to be the key dimensions of modern mortality which are most influenced by contemporary health and social policies. Catastrophic death continues to be massively in evidence at the end of the twentieth century; it is a subject of huge importance to sociological analysis; but it is not one upon which we can concentrate here. Nevertheless, the personal and collective suffering caused by war, famine and natural disasters which are made worse by poverty and inadequate social infrastructures should remain in our minds when we are considering the more 'routine' aspects of modern death. It is a characteristic of modernity that even in the circumscribed and carefully constructed 'peace' of the hospice, the horrors of other forms of death can never be far away.

At the same time the dying process also has its mundane aspects. It may create dependencies, complicating reliance on others, deepening the level of daily physical and personal contact between a dying person and those doing the caring. It may limit personal and practical horizons in a context where social death (Mulkay 1993) further compounds the physical dimensions of dying. Social death in this sense is the experience of becoming of diminishing importance to the lives and concerns of other people, no longer an active participant in the affairs of daily life and therefore someone whose rights and dignity are, by implication, threatened. Death may be experienced as sheer hard work – as the illness advances and as the burdens of caring grow; but it may also be experienced as an opportunity – for personal development or fulfilment in relationships with others. So this book will look at what is known about these issues from a sociological perspective.

In his wide-ranging discussion of aspects of death in contemporary culture, Walter (1994) has produced a helpful typology in which he distinguishes between three characteristic forms of death: *traditional*, *modern* and '*neo-modern*' or '*post-modern*'. These ideal types are of course simplified notions about social life. They have a logical coherence, though they do not exist in their pure form in the world itself. Their value is heuristic – they help us to find out more, to ask the right questions, to discover. In constructing them Walter distinguishes important shifts in the way death can be perceived and organized, and most importantly from a sociological point of view, anchors these in specific historical and social contexts.

Within *traditional* culture death is more a problem for those who survive than for those who are dying. Frequent deaths associated with high infant mortality and low life expectancy constitute a continual threat to the fabric of society. Complex rituals are typical responses to this and are well documented in the anthropological literature (van Gennep 1960). These elaborate rituals provide opportunities for the needs of the group to be reasserted in the face of death. They demonstrate continuity by marking formally the ending of a life and relocating survivors in new positions in the social structure (the son who inherits the responsibilities of the father; the brother-in-law who provides shelter to his dead brother's wife; the widow who goes to live in the family of her husband). They also highlight and reinforce the continuities between the worlds of the living and the dead – by setting aside sacred burial places, by revealing the world of the spirits.

Such responses to death are made possible by (and also help to reinforce) the existence of an overarching system of beliefs and values which characterizes what it means to be a member of this particular culture. These responses to death are typical of societies exhibiting what Durkheim (1933) called 'mechanical solidarity' – where there is a highly developed collective consciousness, where there is an integrated moral framework of shared beliefs and sentiments which binds individuals to the group, and where there is a generally low level of individualization. The authority of religion is paramount here and provides a coherent 'sacred canopy' (Berger 1973) which overarches the social world and which is interpreted on the ground by priests or other religious leaders. Walter suggests that the archetypal death in this context is likely to result from infectious disease such as plague, be rapid in its course and associated with low life expectancy. But even in our own society until recent times glimpses of such traditional aspects of death have been visible. Fieldwork in the Yorkshire fishing village of Staithes (Clark 1982, 1993a) showed a society in which collective representations of grief and mourning were well developed, were rooted in local religious and occupational cultures and, despite some more recent influences from the wider context, were generally robust in character.

Modern death has rather different hallmarks. It is located in societies which observe radical divisions between the public and private dimensions of social life and where family relationships are perceived to be a prime site of individual identity. Here death is associated increasingly with old age, is often hidden from view and is above all understood as both a process and an event which is managed by medical experts. In modernity the archetypal death is from cancer and is regarded as predictable in its course and amenable to clinical interventions, particularly those relating to pain control. When death occurs, however, it is likely to elicit only attenuated ritual responses: it is seen as something that must be 'dealt with' efficiently, quietly and without undue elaboration. In contrast to traditional societies, the disposal of the dead in this context is most usually by cremation, rather than burial. Death as 'taboo' is inextricably linked therefore to the conditions of modernity.

Post-modern death is more elusive, less easy to characterize and can be seen as an emergent aspect of the times in which we are now living. It continues to incorporate some facets of modern death, but with notable elaborations and departures. Thus neo- or post-modern death places greater emphasis on living with dying (rather than the control of death); it is associated with long-term degenerative conditions that may continue into advanced age; but it also has other representations in the form of the new diseases of late modernity, notably AIDS. The surrounding social structure is also subtly different in character: private and public are seen in dynamic interplay, whilst identities are pluralized and subject to reflexive redrafting as the project of the self is caught up in a shifting matrix of relationships which are no longer bounded by the parameters of community or family (we discuss this in more detail in the next section). In this context individuals may seek to assert their own will over the dying process, rejecting the authority of medicine and health care and seeking to assert personal values and meanings. For those who are bereaved there may be counsellors or self-help groups available to offer support, where once the help of neighbours and kin may have sufficed. Death as a meaningful process and as the final stage of some inner psychological journey are characteristics of 'post-modernity'. The consequent rituals at funerals and in memorial services will therefore reflect personal achievements and goals, but express these idiosyncratically through individualized cultural forms and items relevant to the life of the dead person. Post-modern death is therefore likely to result in funerary rituals which reflect the cultural diversity of the times: green, feminist, gay, and so on.

Walter argues that in distinguishing *traditional*, *modern* and *post-modern* death we must give attention to several key dimensions: the bodily context; the social context; the system of authority; notions of coping; the varying concepts of death as a journey; as well as the prevailing values and beliefs associated with death at any given juncture. Although, as he acknowledges, these three types do relate to fairly distinct historical periods, aspects of each can also exist co-terminously. Immigrant groups may maintain traditional elements within an otherwise modern death culture, which nevertheless can also produce neo- or post-modern variations. Within the same society generational or social class differences may likewise reflect aspects of the individual ideal types. Ultimately, Walter seems to suggest that each ideal type does replace the previous one, in historical sequence. The collapse of traditional aspects of death and dying is therefore intimately linked to the rise of modernity which introduced rationalizing systems, undermined communal forms and values, and was profoundly secularizing in character. Efficiency, medicalization, the removal of lay control, have all been objects of criticism within the modern management of death. Death in late modernity however has become increasingly malleable in an individualistic, consumerist culture. Yet Walter acknowledges,

> The trouble with this neo-modern solution, however, is its extreme subjectivity, its radical centring of everything on the self, which then finds itself denied the shelter of the traditional canopy of religion and the modern canopy of medicine.
>
> (Walter 1994: 64)

As we shall see later, it is certain aspects of these modern/post-modern tensions that are at the heart of some current dilemmas in palliative care. They are also central to constructions of identity and the body and to representations of suffering in society.

Identity and the body

During the early 1990s the sociologist Anthony Giddens turned his attention to the relationship between late modernity and the concept of identity, focusing in particular on the reflexive ordering and reordering of social relations (Giddens 1991, 1992). Giddens argues for a notion of 'the self' as a reflexive project, which involves trading off rewards and satisfactions against a shifting array of risks and insecurities. A principal determinant of this reflexive self in modernity is the growth of 'abstract systems' (Giddens 1990) which deskill, alienate and fragment the self; such systems are found, for example, in complex organizations, in the work of professionals and in the achievements of science and technology.

This concept of the self as a fragile project has of course been articulated by other social theorists in recent decades, including Berger and associates (Berger and Luckmann 1971; Berger 1973; Berger et al. 1973; Sennett 1977; Lasch 1980). The significant area of new development however is in the connection between these ideas and the current interest in the sociology of the body. There has been a marked turnaround from the situation in the mid-1980s when Turner (1984) could draw attention to the 'missing body' within sociological concerns. Interest in the sociology of the body has increased dramatically in the interim (Frank 1990; Turner 1992; Scott and Morgan 1993). As a result, possibilities now exist for the introduction of ideas about the body into a number of substantive areas of enquiry, not least Turner's own twin concerns with the sociology of religion and the sociology of health and illness.

Giddens provides an important bridging point between sociologies of 'the self' and of 'the body'. Crucially, for Giddens, the reflexive self is also an *embodied* self. Within late modernity the images, surfaces and experiences of the body become central to conceptions of the self, most obviously in areas such as fashion, dieting and fitness, but more crucially in 'fateful moments' relating to death or sexuality, when the smooth workings of abstract systems are called into question. As a consequence, Giddens argues, sickness and death have become *sequestrated* in modern society, so that death is routinely hidden from view and medicalized. A parallel is drawn here with the removal of sex 'behind the scenes', which Giddens suggests is 'not so much a prurient concealment from view as a reconstituting of sexuality and its refocusing on an emerging sphere of intimacy' (1991: 164). In rather different ways, therefore, both sex and death become entwined in the reflexive project of the self and in the sphere of intimate life but are in turn both present and absent from wider social relations.

Following Giddens, Shilling (1993) gives examples of increasing emphasis on the body in recent times, including the growing interest in self-care in health. He also shows that investment in the body has its limitations, since of course there are biological boundaries to the social construction and

reconstruction of the body. Disease, pain, physical decline, although medi-
ated by social and historical circumstances, pose challenges to the body-as-
project. As Shilling notes, Bauman (1992) has seen recent self-care projects
as specific attempts to overcome the body's limitations and in so doing
deny the broader challenge which is posed by the biological irreducibility
of the body.

What all this serves to emphasize is the important role which the body
has in the reflexive ordering of identity. Bourdieu's contribution to this
(Bourdieu 1984), as Shilling points out, is the notion of 'physical capital',
whereby the body is seen to create and possess value in certain social fields.
Featherstone (1987) has noted the relevance of the ageing process to this
and the related social class dimensions. He suggests that, while working-
class people, as they grow older, may come to accept the body as, in some
sense, a machine in decline, members of the new middle classes may experience the deterioration of the 'body-as-project' as a source of acute anxiety.
In the upper classes, by contrast, visible signs of ageing are worn unself-
consciously as a mark of status. Similarly, Hepworth (1984) has pointed
out some of the key gender differences in the ageing process which are
constructed and managed differently for men and women, not least as they
relate to perceptions of sexuality and physical attractiveness. Shilling highlights the importance of all this for a sociological understanding of death:

> I view death as having become a particular existential problem for
> people as a result of modern forms of embodiment, rather than being
> a universal problem for human beings which assumes the same form
> irrespective of time and place.
>
> (Shilling 1993: 177)

A pattern may be discerned here in which the *future prospect* of death
becomes of central concern to us all. This is 'living with dying', and is
characterized by the preponderance of death in old age, the early diagnosis
of life-threatening disease, the prolongation of illness trajectories, and active
intervention by professionals in the dying process. Such interventions are
most clearly seen in the activities of medical and health care specialists, but
are also visible in the current preoccupation of private individuals to avoid
untimely death or the exacerbation of a pre-existing condition by means of
careful attention to bodily signs, nutrition and 'fitness': both physical and
emotional. Society thus becomes organized on the basis of avoiding the
risk of death:

> Death is a momentary event, but defence of health and vigilance
> against its enemies is a life-long labour. Death comes at the end of life,
> defence of health fills the whole of it. The price for exchanging immor-
> tality for health is life lived in the shadow of death; to postpone death,
> one needs to surrender life to fighting it.
>
> (Bauman 1992: 20)

In this patterning of ideas the long journey towards death is seen as not only a threat, but also an opportunity to reach personal fulfilment and development of self. Kübler-Ross's powerful conceptual image of death as the final stage of growth (1975) has been particularly influential in this characterization. Seen in this context, death in late modernity is caught up in wider discourses – of identity, of the body, and of the nature of suffering itself.

Representations of suffering

Discussions about the changing construction of the body and about the potential for death to become sequestrated in late modernity point to some far-reaching changes, occurring over the last 200 years. By the late eighteenth century, with the age of modernization gathering momentum, European bourgeois society had begun to experience a growing sense of optimism and confidence about notions of progress and social improvement. Despite political unrest, revolutions and mass migration, these ideas were increasingly the hallmark of nineteenth-century European culture. It was an optimism which saw few limits to human ascendancy over the natural world. Medicine, of course, was no exception to this process and the nineteenth century saw a growing emphasis upon scientific discovery and medical ascendancy coupled with the great programme of hospital building, particularly in the large cities.

At the start of the twenty-first century, however, we appear as a society less confident in the principles of social progress and unproblematic advancement. Rather the contemporary attitude is infused with profound doubt about the status of scientific knowledge. Such knowledge appears open to chronic, incessant revision in the light of new 'discoveries' and 'breakthroughs'. This in turn is coupled to growing environmental concerns about the unintended consequences of scientific 'progress'. Doubts of this kind are also linked to a pervasive sense of mistrust in the role of experts and the activities of professionals, so that individuals may see themselves as weighing and judging the relative 'risks' of following one set of advice, as opposed to another. This of course has its correlates in a consumer culture where health care, religion and bodily regimens may somehow be seen as part of a range of lifestyle options to be selected or rejected at will. In such a context individual 'needs', preferences and choices may be seen to predominate over those of community, collectivity or society. It is therefore in this framework that we must think about representations of suffering in society, not as some fixed sub-stratum which shapes a common experience, but rather as something dynamic and fluid in character, influenced profoundly by social context.

Sociology should have something to offer here. Its preoccupations with questions of agency and structure, the relationship between the individual and society, and the forces of social change, all allow it to contribute a view on the changing construction of suffering. One formulation is to consider suffering at three conceptual levels: individual, social and societal, and to examine the relationships between these.

At the *individual* level, attention is drawn to the personal encounter with suffering in the uniquely bounded experience of one person. Making sense of suffering at this level involves understanding personal reactions to discomfort, distress, disorder and disease. It may be the case here that individual explanations of suffering are important and these may focus around personal *theodicies*: Why me? Why now? Why like this? We can identify here a territory which might be labelled the spirituality of suffering and where individuals may be able to forge, for themselves, some meaning to aspects of their existence, located through the experience of distress. That individuals should do this *ab initio* is itself a rather modern concept and reflects the high levels of individualism which characterize contemporary social life. The study of these areas may allow us to establish some kind of phenomenology of suffering. This might show the necessary and sufficient conditions for the existence of suffering, not as defined by 'experts', but rather from the perspectives of suffering individuals themselves. Or it may further persuade us that suffering must always be relative, bounded by context and expectations and resistant to easy generalization.

Sociologists have contributed a great deal in recent years to understanding suffering in this way and we now have some fine studies, particularly in the area of chronic illness, which highlight the importance of personal meanings, biographical factors and lay beliefs in shaping the individual experience of sickness (for a review, see Bury 1991). By focusing on the words and accounts of individuals this work has highlighted the value of illness narratives as a course of understanding. A particularly interesting perspective on these issues has been developed by the Canadian sociologist, Arthur Frank. Drawing upon his own personal experience of heart disease and cancer, coupled with an interest in post-modern ideas, he suggests that ill people have a powerful need to tell stories of their experience. In this way they are able to 'construct new maps and new perceptions of their relationship to the world' (1995: 3). The *embodiment* of these stories is also important, for as Frank puts it: 'they are told not just about the body, but through it' (1995: 3). From this perspective he is able to identify three particular narratives of illness. In the *restitution narrative*, the active player is the remedy, the triumph of medicine, the magic bullet: today I am ill, but tomorrow I will be well again, thanks to this treatment, that new idea, some revolutionary new drug. This is the narrative of modernity and as such it has profound limitations when it collides with the realization of mortality; for when death becomes inevitable, there is no story left to tell. In the *chaos narrative* the voice of the teller becomes lost in the disorganization of suffering; the paradigmatic case for this is probably Alzheimer's

Disease. 'Chaos stories', Frank observes, 'are as anxiety provoking as restitution stories are preferred' (1995: 97). *Quest narratives* however meet
suffering head on; they afford ill persons their most distinctive voice. They
involve a sense of illness as a journey, they recognize ill people as responsible moral agents and they serve to restore a sense of moral agency which
is lost in the narratives of restitution and chaos.

Just such a quest narrative can be seen in Brodsky's (1995) study of men
who had suffered from and 'survived' testicular cancer. Again, researching
the subject following his own experience of the illness, Brodsky found
among those he interviewed four key impacts. First, the men reported a
change in what Brodsky calls 'the identification self'; they viewed themselves
and their lives more purposefully. Second, the 'interpersonal self' was
changed and they found themselves capable of more enriching relationships with others. Third, there were negative implications for the 'bodily self',
but this tended to be only a short-term sense of concern about physical
changes caused by the illness. Lastly, the 'achieving self' was altered, and
the men reported reduced interest in matters of personal ambition and a
greater sense of realism about work and life goals.

Individuals are of course social beings and give meaning to their experiences through encounters with others around them, in intimate relationships, in families, social networks, communities, as well as in the context
of formal organizations of various kinds. Suffering at this more explicitly
social level would therefore address itself to a rather wider context. Here
we begin to think about the norms and values which relate to suffering in
society at a particular moment. We start to consider what *should* as well
as what *does* constitute suffering. We also start to move into the realm
of ethics, talking for example of 'senseless suffering', of 'necessary' and
'unnecessary suffering' and 'avoidable' suffering. Such terms contribute to
what we might call a *moral order* of suffering. This implies that suffering is not a uniform currency of equal exchange value. It may well be that
the suffering of one person is somehow deemed more 'tragic', 'worthy' or
'shameful' than that of another. Such debates are frequently taken up in
the popular press, where they can polarize opinion or fuel prejudice against
marginal groups in society. Examples which spring to mind include the
debates around resource allocation for people infected with HIV, or the
example in a Welsh hospice in 1997 of the remand prisoner who up to just
a few hours before his life ended had to be kept chained to his bed, on the
instruction of prison authorities.

Traditionally, the codification of moral orders has been an important
domain for organized religion and each of the world religions has some
form of theological framework for the explanation of suffering in the
world. Around the globe, these teachings continue to hold sway for many
millions of people. In the West, however, where Christian religious traditions have predominated, the picture has become highly complex (Bruce

1996). Simple measures, such as church membership and church attendance, show unequivocal evidence of a decline in religiosity. A belief in some of the elements of formal religion however seems rather more persistent and it is certainly the case that among some groups – evangelicals, members of cults, sects and other new religious movements – there is evidence of a powerful influence of religious teaching on everyday life. Some individuals may therefore ignore more personal and idiosyncratic explanations of suffering in a context where a clearly defined framework of overarching belief is in place. In general however, for most Westerners, theology, belief, ritual and religious teaching emanating from the churches represent only one source of ideas about the meaning and purpose of suffering and no longer constitute the entire perspective on the subject.

Finally, the social dimension of suffering is shaped through the role of formal organizations, particularly the professions within the medical division of labour. The nineteenth and twentieth centuries have seen the increasing refinement and differentiation of this division of labour as new professions, such as physiotherapy, occupational therapy, dietetics and speech and language therapy have emerged. At the same time nursing and medicine have become increasingly differentiated internally, with numerous areas of sub-specialty. Debates continue of course (Turner 1996) over the extent to which medicine has been successful in maintaining dominance over its colleague health professions. Within medicine however there is a growing acknowledgement of its failure to respond fully to the nature of human suffering, coupled with a recognition of the limits of biomedicine. As the physician Eric J. Cassell puts it in the opening lines of his book on the nature of suffering:

> The test of a system of medicine should be its adequacy in the face of suffering; this book starts from the premise that modern medicine fails that test.
>
> (Cassell 1991: vii)

This brings us to an appreciation of suffering at what we might term the *societal* level. Here we move away to some extent from the territory of meanings, norms and values. We now begin to focus on complex patterns and distributions of health-related suffering. Interestingly, these are again expressed through different disciplines, such as epidemiology and demography. We are addressing here the highest level of the social organization of suffering, through areas of health policy, government strategy and political economy. These we will turn to in more detail later in the book. They suggest that we have arrived at the level of what might be called *aggregated suffering*, where individual experiences and values become less central than those of the collectivity or of society as a whole. At this level processes of governance become the mechanism for determining how suffering is to be relieved. Attention now focuses on what can be invested, what strategies pursued, what services developed and what measures of success may be applied against these.

Dying in late modern culture

In the middle years of this century, during the post-Second World War era, death fell into the now recognizable pattern of being predominantly an expected, anticipated event at the end of a prolonged period of old age. The recognition that peacetime dying and mourning had become despiritualized, secularized and medicalized spawned a number of empirical studies. Some of these focused on the individual expression, experience and resolution of the 'sickness' of grief (Lindemann 1944; Marris 1958; Gorer 1965).

The central theme in these empirical studies and in other 'classic' texts on grief (Freud 1913; Bowlby 1980; Raphael 1984; Murray Parkes 1986) is that grieving leads to the detachment of the survivor from the dead person, and a formation of new attachments. The journey through grief leads the sufferer through various strong emotions, with a resulting resolution of anger, guilt, depression and sadness. In 'normal grief' a point of emotional equilibrium is achieved in which the sufferer accepts what has happened and moves on to new relationships and affectional bonds. One particularly influential concept that has emerged from the literature on the individual response to grief is that of 'anticipatory grief' (Lindemann 1944), where mourning takes place in anticipation of the event of death. It has been used predominantly as an explanatory tool in studies of the reactions of people and their families who are dealing with terminal cancer (Rando 1986). As a consequence of its influence in this field, it has been assumed to be a useful construct for exploring experiences associated with other life-limiting conditions (Fulton *et al.* 1996). However the trajectory of non-cancer conditions is often very different from that associated with cancer. The 'living–dying' interval is prolonged, and punctuated by fluctuations in the condition. Relapse and reprieve alternate, and deterioration is both slow and difficult to recognize. Anticipation of death is replaced by the repeated experience of, and 'present grief' for, multiple, smaller losses (Pattison 1978; Garner 1997).

When applied to the experience of dying, these concepts of the processual nature of grief encourage the dying person to assume a particular role of 'modern dying' (Field 1996). In this role, 'heroism' is relocated in a range of socially sanctioned behaviours all of which are directed at the inward adaptation of the psyche to the threat of death. Appropriate behaviours become less important than the confessional of self to others, and the wresting of control over the manner of dying. This celebration of individualism occurs when the dying person becomes aware of his or her prognosis and 'collaborates' with health care professionals to make choices which are consistent with individual beliefs about the right way to die.

As Williams points out, the development of the modern hospice movement under the leadership of Cicely Saunders gave these ideas widespread credence and gave a new meaning to the concept of 'ritual dying' (1990: 121). Seale's analysis of survey data (1995), undertaken as part of a larger study (Seale and Cartwright 1994) concerned with experiences during the last year of life, shows empirically how such discourses have permeated the public consciousness. He traces the attribution of 'heroism' to the deaths of others within the narrative accounts of their dying, as given by their close companions. The basis of heroism is portrayed by respondents as:

> . . . a struggle against external and internal enemies to gain knowledge, the opportunity to demonstrate courage and a beatific state in which 'carers' and dying people participate. Unlike more traditional forms of heroism, this script deviates from celebrating solely masculine qualities and includes a female heroics of care, concern and emotional expression.
>
> (Seale 1995: 597)

Both Seale (1995) and Field (1996) suggest however that the 'modern role of dying' based on awareness, self-determination and this type of reflexive heroism is not available to those large sections of the community who die slowly from old age and chronic conditions not readily labelled as 'terminal':

> The dominance of the discourse of awareness, however, poses certain problems for individuals who cannot be scripted into the drama. The forms of dying that are most amenable for inclusion into the heroic script of aware dying are those from cancer and AIDS. In these deaths, dramatic moments of truth are reached and either confronted or avoided . . . Those who die in extreme old age, however, the demented and the institutionalised have much less opportunity to strike a heroic pose, but are more frequently portrayed as dribbling undignified figures waiting for death as a release from life . . .
>
> (Seale 1995: 612)

Part of the romantic appeal of the modern way of dying is an emphasis on community and 'home' as the best place within which to end one's life. Current preoccupations with the availability of home deaths confirms the strength of this notion. Institutionalized death is seen as a second best option to the more 'natural' death at home. In a paper based on the larger survey referred to above Seale (1990) points out that home death may not be a realistic option for some older people. There are two reasons for this: first, they may lack an informal carer on whom home-based care largely depends and, second, a point of clear transition between being 'ill' and 'dying' will be lacking in many non-cancer conditions. For this group, death may come suddenly during what has been assumed to be yet another acute exacerbation of an underlying chronic condition. A further aspect of the romanticism of the modern role of dying is the almost mythical hero-ism associated with the 'battle' against pain. Several studies have revealed pain as the most universally feared symptom of the cancer death (Dent and Goulston 1982; Levine *et al.* 1985; Foley 1993), in spite of long-standing expert evidence that such pain can be well controlled in almost all cases (Twycross and Lack 1983). Deaths from conditions other than cancer are not always afforded this particular badge of honour. Rather, death creeps up painlessly, slowly and with increasing mental and physical infirmity.

Williams (1990) suggests that the picture may be more complex than the straightforward assumption of ideas which stem from the contemporary hegemony of professional deathwork discourse. Based on the analysis of a series of in-depth qualitative interviews with older people in Aberdeen and the results of a larger scale questionnaire survey, he found that individuals interweave cultural ideas about dying and bereavement from various his-torical influences. In this process potentially paradoxical ideas are com-bined actively according to personal circumstances and previous experiences of deaths. Williams identified clear patterns in these ideas about dying, describing a preference among one group of respondents for 'ritual dying' which combined a value on achieving readiness for death with an emphasis on the reunion of the dying with those close to them. A second group expressed a preference for 'disregarded' dying. This combined the moral expectation of death in old age with the ideal of a quick and unaware death. A third group of respondents exhibited a pattern of what Williams calls 'transitional' ideas about death. Here, elements of ritual and dis-regarded dying are combined. A minority in Williams' study expressed a preference for 'controlled' dying in which the ordering of one's fate was paramount. This latter group feared both pain and increasing dependency, and saw euthanasia or suicide as a real option in avoiding these states.

We have tried to show then, in this first chapter, how the experiences of suffering and dying have essentially sociological characteristics. Whilst they appeal to some of the most fundamental aspects of human existence, we can also see that there is little irreducibility about suffering and dying. The distinction between traditional, modern and post-modern death is particu-larly helpful in this regard and opens up our thinking to the changing historical and social constructions of death and dying. We have begun to focus upon some of the particular characteristics of suffering and dying within contemporary, late modern culture and already we have a sense of some of the particular features which are in evidence. We begin to see something of the importance of narratives of illness and dying, not just as stories about physical and mental suffering, but as tales which are told through the body itself. In the next chapter we develop these ideas in a little more detail with particular reference to ageing, the experience of informal care giving and processes of bereavement.

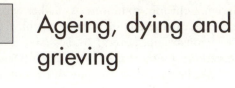

2 Ageing, dying and grieving

We have already alluded to the case which has been made for seeing the study of death as central to the sociological enterprise. In this chapter we hope to reinforce this point by showing how death and dying touch on at least two sub-specialties of social science research which, though they may be reluctant to acknowledge it, are of major importance to death studies. We are referring here to the study of human ageing and to that area of work which focuses on the experience of informal care giving to sick and dependent people.

At various points in the book we shall be arguing for greater attention to the links between ageing and death. In this we have no wish to ignore deaths in infancy, childhood or mid-life; simply we seek to acknowledge that within contemporary culture, death for most comes at the end of a long life. For these reasons the ways in which we think about the care of dying people cannot be divorced from the question of how we think about the care of older people more generally, and the place they occupy in society.

For similar reasons, the debates about informal care – about the experience of caring for a dependent person, and about the policy implications of this – cannot be separated from the reality that those receiving this care will also die. Again however it is a characteristic of the narrow focus of those who study 'the care of the dying', or who provide services to dying people and their informal carers, that they often overlook the longer term nature of the caring biography. The needs of 'informal carers' do not suddenly become an issue when the persons for whom they are caring are suddenly designated as 'dying'. Indeed a variety of organizations may already have been involved, perhaps even over many years, in assisting with such needs. So understanding informal care at the end of life must be rooted in what we know about informal care in other contexts and settings, and we try to illustrate this here.

For many informal carers, who themselves are likely to be older people, the experience of bereavement is widespread. Where this takes place in the context of married couples, we need again to recognize the wider social circumstances. Debates on the high levels of divorce in contemporary culture often overlook the fact that modern marriages are far likelier to endure for half a century or more than ever they were in the past (Clark and Haldane 1990). So spouse bereavement, when it occurs, may be after many years of marriage, presenting a lengthy and accumulated personal script of experiences which are thrown into sharp relief by the loss. The meaning of such bereavements must surely be different from those following other relationships, less protracted in character. Helpfully, we have evidence that bereavement theorists are willing to look to changing social and cultural factors in making sense of individual losses, a field which until recently has been heavily dominated by psychological and psycho-dynamic perspectives.

By considering such issues in this chapter we hope to show more fully how the manner of our dying and of our grieving is inextricably intertwined with the manner of our living and our ageing.

Ageing and dying

The gerontologist Victor Marshall has remarked that 'the social sciences have contributed little to our understanding of ageing and dying' (1996: 57). It is the conjunction of the two subjects which is important here, for undoubtedly there is now a large social scientific literature both on aspects of ageing and on matters of death and dying. Gerontology however has placed such a strong emphasis on positive images of the ageing process, on opposing ageism and upon questions of advocacy for older people, that it has seemed incapable at times of acknowledging that the aged also die. Similarly, students of death, dying and bereavement frequently overlook the relationship between their subject matter and the wider context of ageing in society. Yet there are important areas where the two overlap and must necessarily combine as a field of study. In this section we therefore include a brief discussion of debates surrounding the social construction of old age, together with an examination of different theoretical perspectives on ageing. We then return to the work of Marshall on ageing and death as interrelated topics.

Phillipson and Thompson (1996) suggest that three factors have influenced public discussion of old age in recent decades. First, there has been a considerable growth of interest in issues of ageing which has been fuelled in particular by debates about pensions; this of course focuses on how pensions are to be paid for in societies where older people represent a substantial proportion of the population. Second, there is the impact of community care policies upon services for older people. Third, increases in the phenomenon of 'early retirement' have created interest in notions of the 'third age' and later life as a period of extensive opportunities. Each of these, Phillipson and Thompson argue, has served to highlight ways in which old age is *socially constructed*. This means that we cannot adopt a simple biological model of old age as a phase of life in which increasing physical limitation sets the parameters for the level and character of an individual's wider social engagement. Indeed social constructionism in this form challenges a type of biological reductionism which too easily can provide the justification for denying older people their rights. A further dimension of this approach is to emphasize diversity and heterogeneity, thus chronological age is only one variable which might shape individual experience; others will include ethnicity, social class, gender, involvement in the labour market, income, housing. In other words older people must be seen, like their younger counterparts, as *socially differentiated*. Older people may however be constructed as a particular kind of 'problem' within late capitalist societies, where they are associated with poverty and social exclusion and are looked upon as a burden to society as a whole. Conversely, social constructionism can reveal more positive images of ageing, viewing later life as a time for reorientation, with older people active in a search for fulfilment and meaning which involves redefining work, leisure, intimate relationships and friendships. It is clear from this that what constitutes old age, still less 'normal ageing', is by no means a matter for consensus. Old age as a problem for sociology, in terms of how the discipline makes sense of it, constructs and answers questions around it, and promotes a comparative understanding of it, is to some extent revealed in a number of theories of ageing.

Disengagement was seen by Cumming and Henry (1961) as the 'natural' process of withdrawal from society which accompanies ageing, and as such an essential criterion for 'successful' ageing. It is seen to involve a mutual process of declining reciprocity between older people and the wider society, something regarded as essential to and beneficial for the maintenance of a stable social structure. This argument, which is rooted in structural functionalism, has of course been widely criticized (Turner 1987: Chapter 6). It can, for example, be seen to condone policy indifference to the needs of older people, who experience declining material well-being and reduced opportunities in later life; moreover, disengagement may be an involuntary experience, encountered as part of a coercive form of social death.

The converse of disengagement is *activity* theory (Havinghurst 1963), which argues that successful ageing is predicated upon maintaining into old age the activity patterns and values of earlier life, replacing lost networks and contacts as necessary in order to maintain life satisfaction. Again, as Turner (1987) points out, there is a strong whiff of middle-class North

American values to this position, masquerading as something normative for society as a whole. Indeed, for those who lack material resources, attempts to establish and maintain such activity levels may serve to reinforce a sense of isolation and prejudice.

In the United Kingdom, and in contrast to functional theories of ageing, policy analysts have tended to focus more on issues relating to the *political economy of old age*. Thus writers such as Townsend (1981) and Walker (1986) have focused on the configuration of political and economic structures affecting older people in the second half of the twentieth century. This position emphasizes the structural dependency of older people which results from restricted access to resources, especially income. It draws attention to the importance of poverty in later life as something affecting one quarter of older people and shows how society is predicated on rewarding current rather than past work. In contrast to notions of the 'third age' surrounding early retirement, it also points to the ways in which older workers are pushed into unemployment and less skilled jobs and shows how the declining value of savings impacts on the very old.

It is possible in these theories of ageing to identify differing preoccupations and interests. Whether the remedy is disengagement or activity, the underlying concern is with the normalization of old age in order to achieve both a harmonious status passage for the older individual and a societal adjustment which maintains social equilibrium. These approaches therefore draw upon functionalist ideas which place particular emphasis on the interrelatedness of different elements within the social system as a key to stability. Within this framework older people must have a clearly defined place in society, linked to appropriate roles and social expectations. By contrast, ideas which originate in the analysis of structured inequalities point to ways in which older people are disadvantaged within late capitalist systems of production, consumption and welfare. What appears lacking in both of these perspectives are studies which focus on the meanings and interpretations which older people give to their lives and circumstances. How old people regard death and the dying process, their views about what constitutes a 'good death' or about where and in what circumstances they may wish to die, are issues largely absent from the literature.

Some qualitative studies are available however which explore the 'life world' of being old. Thompson *et al.* (1991), for example, looked at the experience of later life, focusing on the disjuncture between the bodily appearance of ageing and perceptions of 'self'. Bamford (1994) explored the life history of 28 men and women who were grandparents, asking them to describe how becoming old had affected their lives, together with their hopes, fears and expectations for the future. A repeated theme in this study was that older people used life experience actively to make sense of, and cope with, the changes wrought by bereavement, retirement and family transition.

Based on a study among older people in Aberdeen, Williams (1990) identified three coherent conceptual patterns of ageing. Some respondents were optimistic, viewing ageing as a 'resurgence' of opportunity and interest; this attitude was seen as a protective way of life, one which could enable long-term resistance to mental confusion and institutionalization. Other respondents viewed old age as a 'siege', in which ageing was associated with a threat to one's social position and defensive action was necessary to avoid becoming 'truly old'. The last, and most prevalent, pattern of ideas identified by Williams was that in which ageing was regarded as a 'delayed capitulation'; this patterning of ideas

> ... included an ultimate pessimism about late old age, a conviction that in the end, for those who lived long enough, it was necessary and legitimate to lay down one's arms and accept the care of others.
>
> (Williams 1990: 77)

Little is known about the experiences or attitudes of those who reach very old age. Bury and Holme (1991) conducted the only British study of late old age, which is based on reports of the lives of 200 people aged over 90 years. The considerable physical constraints placed on the daily lives of very old people are described, but with an emphasis on communicating the diversity and complexity of ageing. Bury and Holme (1991: 163) note the reluctance of very old people to complain about their lives, their stoicism and willingness to accept life as it is. They interpret this as an attitudinal stance learnt by socialization to very firm cultural mores in early life. The values of patience, of 'knowing one's place', and of religious devotion were particularly important to this group.

One of the only studies which has used a large-scale survey methodology to examine views about ageing is the Eurobarometer survey of public attitudes to ageing and older people in the member states of the European Community (Walker 1993). This was an amalgamation of two surveys, one of which charted the views of the general public aged over 15 years; while the other charted the views of older people themselves. The report represents a comprehensive view of ageing from these two potentially very different perspectives. The surveys show that older people prefer to be known as 'senior citizens' rather than any other term. The analysts report that

> ... this seemed to signal some kind of positive statement from this group that they either want to be regarded as people, who just happen to be older than some others, or as citizens like the rest of the community.
>
> (Walker 1993: 7)

This feeling that older people are simply 'people' like everyone else was confirmed by the survey of the younger age groups. They tended not to agree with a statement that older people were due admiration and respect simply for being old. Similarly, older people reported that they had experienced no major changes in life satisfaction as a result of becoming old, nor had their activity levels diminished markedly. Illness and disability did lead to a small reduction in activities, while the onset of the 'fourth' age at 75+ was associated with a significant decline in activity. Only a small proportion of older people perceived that they had ever been treated as second-class citizens, but on the occasions when this had happened, public agencies and politicians were reported as groups most likely to discriminate. Older people tended to live alone, but to maintain close ties with their families. The authors of the report note that the term 'intimacy at a distance' (Rosenmayer and Kockeis 1963) captures perfectly the perceived links between older people and their families. However, loneliness was perceived as a problem, and further, older people tended to agree with a statement put to them which suggested that families are less likely to be willing to care for older relatives. This was in spite of evidence from the survey of the general population which suggested that this statement is a 'modern myth'. Among older people, independence was perceived as an important value and a strong preference was expressed for staying at home with the support, if necessary, of 'home care' provided by the state. Financially, older people perceived themselves as relatively secure, but only by dint of care being exerted over expenditure. While strong support was voiced for the 'social contract' by the general population, in most countries the state pension was perceived as inadequate by older people. This was linked to a frustration of aspirations and feelings of resentment.

Finally, we must acknowledge that a great deal of attention has focused on the demographics of old age, and for the most part within Western societies, this is constructed as a problem. Warnes (1996) has provided a clear and thoughtful review of this complex and contentious area. He begins by pointing out that the principal reason for increased life expectancy in the twentieth century is the fall in infant mortality, rather than major improvements in mortality in later life, though survival rates in old age are increasing. The declining death rate on both sides of the Atlantic has two possible causes: the fall in infectious diseases and general improvements in public health, coupled with the changing character of medical intervention. Fertility rates also have an impact upon the age structure of the population. Low rates of fertility create a large share in the elderly population, which characterizes the modern West.

As Warnes points out, such trends contribute to public anxieties about the expanding elderly population, creating fears of a demographic 'time bomb', and concern about the massive problem of dependency which will result. We should however be cautious about such rhetoric, not only on moral grounds, but also in relation to the evidence itself.

Writing specifically about the United Kingdom context, Warnes observes:

A detail meriting wider dissemination is that during the 1980s the population in Great Britain aged 60–69 years decreased by 43,000. That fall, associated with fewer births during the 1910s compared to the first decade of the century, will manifest itself during the 1990s among people in their seventies, and during the first decade of the next century among those in their eighties. It is true that there will be a resurgence of elderly population growth from around 2005 for two decades, as the high birth cohorts of the period 1945–1965 reach 60 years of age. But few accounts trace the connection between the records of birth and the fluctuating number achieving old age. Instead, the tendency is to present demographic ageing as a boundless prospect.

(Warnes 1996: 32)

So by taking the longer view this 'boundless' growth in the numbers and proportion of elderly people in society is called into question. In this way fear of a 'tidal wave' of elderly people can be exposed as an ideological construction fuelled alternately by those seeking to reduce the costs of state support in old age and those seeking to obtain greater resources for the relevant services.

Viewed in terms of this discussion, the disjuncture of the ageing literature from that on death and dying becomes all the more baffling. In late modern societies it is ageing, *par excellence*, which precedes death for the large majority of individuals, regardless of class, gender, ethnicity or location. Of course, within these social parameters ageing may take many forms and in so doing will contribute to the diverse social manifestations of death within late modern culture. To study the two interrelatedly therefore has a good deal to offer.

Marshall (1996) sets out some ideas for the generation of theoretical statements and propositions about this relationship between ageing and dying. He begins by suggesting that changing demographics give death a greater predictability, making it something now most likely to occur at the end of a fully completed life course. Returning to Walter's (1993) distinction between traditional, modern and post-modern death, we can see an important transformation here. Deaths of old people, which are anticipated and have greater predictability, have very different implications for the social order from those deaths which occur suddenly at earlier stages of life. Deaths among older people may well be constructed as more of a problem at the level of the individual than at the level of society. Even though they may occur in large numbers they create no substantive threat to the social or moral order. Rather, their impact is local and individualized. They relate particularly to the reflexive project of the self, where death must be given meaning in the context of an individual's completed life course, and constructed as an unproblematic ending.

The difficulty with this position arises from the fact that, as Marshall points out, 'contemporary dying takes longer' (1996: 60). In this sense it is the *dying process*, rather than death itself which is problematic for elderly people, as they, those close to them and their professional carers seek to make sense of events and circumstances at the end of life. Giddens captures this in a passage on the sequestration of death.

> Death remains the great extrinsic factor of human existence; it cannot as such be brought within the internally referential systems of modernity. However, all types of event leading up to and involved with the process of dying can be so incorporated.
>
> (Giddens 1991: 162)

As we shall see in later chapters, the internally referential systems associated with hospice and palliative care have done a great deal to colonize this territory and in so doing to forge a connection between processes of ageing and of dying. Indeed, Marshall (1996) suggests that care institutions are likely to be particularly important sources of cultural meanings relating to ageing and death.

So, following Marshall, one general proposition on the connection between ageing and death which we might derive relates to the impact of changing demographics on the process of dying. We might formulate this as follows: where life expectancy is increased and the highest rates of mortality occur in advanced years, then the social implications of death are likely to be greater at the individual than at the societal level. A correlate of this will be an extended period of dying which is likely to be colonized by professional ideologies, practices and organizations associated with the provision of care to the aged dying, who also pronounce on the meanings and values which surround death among elderly people.

Marshall's second set of statements focuses on the social implications of what he calls 'awareness of finitude' (1996: 69) – the recognition that one's time to death may be limited and death may be growing nearer. This awareness begins to increase in the middle years; it may become more marked when individuals pass the ages at which their own parents died, and also as members of a peer group begin to die. These external markers may be accompanied by changes in individual perception of health status, and recognition of reduced mobility or physical capacity. Marshall sees a psychological dimension to these processes which expresses itself in orientation to time; the future assumes somewhat less importance, the past becomes rather more significant. Here is the phenomenon of 'life review' in which attempts may be made to construct a meaningful narrative where elements of the individual biography are legitimated in some coherent whole. These reminiscence activities may be perceived in a positive way for those involved and they may be encouraged by health and social care professionals; but they may also be accompanied by darker psychological experiences. As Marshall puts it, 'Heightened awareness of finitude leads to increased concerns about the meaning of death itself' (1996: 69). In the absence, however, of any formal religious beliefs on this question, attention may turn to a search for personal control over the dying process.

So from this we might derive a second general proposition: as the life course advances, individuals become increasingly aware of their own finitude; this is likely to promote processes of reflexive life review and the legitimation of biography. Difficulties in giving meaning to death itself however are likely to result in the desire to exercise control over the dying process.

It can be seen from this that both of the propositions we have derived result in an emphasis on control of dying. In late modernity, and at the end of a long life, death is less likely to be reached in the confidence of religious faith. Instead it stands as a feared inconvenience, something less likely to evoke profound existential doubt than as a barrier to the successful completion of the life review process. Woody Allen's oft-quoted 'I don't fear death, it's just that I don't want to be around when it happens' neatly encapsulates this late modern disposition. So it may be that elderly people in Western cultures will seek further influence on how they die, driven by a desire to contextualize this as the appropriate ending to a long life, but rather less preoccupied with explaining the significance of their own mortality in transcendent terms. Such an approach, which sees ageing, dying and death through the reflexive filter of late modernity, presents a number of challenges for those involved in empirical studies of this subject matter.

Informal care

David Field and others (Field *et al.* 1995) have pointed out that, to date, much research-based knowledge about the experience of dying in late modern societies comes only indirectly through the experiences and views of others, chiefly kin or professional carers. Narratives of dying, as produced by dying people themselves, are surprisingly rare in the research literature. A good deal of debate has therefore ensued about the validity of such surrogate or proxy viewpoints (Cartwright and Seale 1990; Spiller and Alexander 1993; Higginson, Priest and McCarthy 1994; Hinton 1996). Attention has focused, for example, around such questions as whether terminally ill people and their carers share an 'open awareness context' in which each is able to acknowledge the fact of dying (Ahmedzai *et al.* 1988), or which group reports higher levels of symptoms and problems (Cartwright and Seale 1990; Spiller and Alexander 1993). In the study reported by Field and colleagues (1995) 28 matched pairs of patients newly admitted to an in-patient hospice were interviewed, together with their informal carers. In common with other studies it was found that informal carers reported higher levels of psychological distress and physical symptoms in the sick person than did the sick people themselves. Carers also tended to overestimate the patients' awareness of their condition. There was however a high level of agreement on satisfaction with the professional care received. Field and colleagues conclude that informal carers are a reliable-within-limits proxy for patients' own views, but aver strongly to studies which directly involve the latter, where this is ethically and practically possible.

Perhaps a more productive line of enquiry from a sociological point of view is to adopt the position taken by Seale (1995a, b) who, following Hammersley (1992), argues that accounts of dying generated by informal carers have two dimensions. First, they can be treated as *topics*, in which the speaker or person being interviewed is provided with an opportunity to present a particular aspect or version of experience. Second, they can be regarded as *resources* for discovering the perspective of the dying or dead person. In the first category the accounts are seen as sociologically problematic – what do they tell us about the social or cultural situation; in what circumstances is such an account possible? In the second, they are regarded as data which, despite certain biases, allow us access to a particular situation.

It is clear from this discussion that understanding the dilemmas, needs and circumstances of the dying person is intricately bound up with those who are providing care, particularly kin, neighbours and friends. Until recently such people, often referred to as 'informal carers', have generally been overlooked in social and policy analysis. As Twigg and Atkin (1994) show, two factors have increased the visibility of informal carers. First, feminist scholars have pointed to the importance of understanding the gendered nature of informal care and the ways in which it relates to assumptions and expectations of women's roles in families. Second, within social policy there has been a growing interest in the activities of informal carers, rooted in their potential contribution to wider aspects of 'care in the community' as a policy goal. As Neale (1991) points out in a review of informal care provided to terminally ill people, informal care giving is an activity encompassing a wide spectrum, from social and psychological support through to the intimate physical care of a sick and dependent person. It may well run the gamut of activities which in other contexts are undertaken by individual and specialized professionals, such as social workers, nurses, doctors and counsellors. Informal carers may provide practical help, like cleaning, cooking and shopping; they may administer drugs, give baths, deal with problems of incontinence, as well as listen, advise and reassure.

'Caring' in this way has been identified as both the range of activities involved in giving personal aid and support to someone in need, *and* the emotions associated with an interpersonal relationship. Graham's description of caring as 'a labour of love' (1983) captures succinctly the way in which care activities are interpreted as evidence of affective ties between people, especially where those involved are related by kinship. The terms 'caring' and 'carer' became a particular focus of analytical attention in the 1980s and 1990s. The history of policy statements concerning the provision of care for sick and dependent people in the second half of the twentieth century.may be seen as a changing configuration of emphasis on the appropriate use and combination of statutory, voluntary and family sources, but in which a fundamental reliance has been placed on family care. This reliance has been couched both as a matter of financial necessity *and* a matter of the preservation of deeply held common values about the obligations of kinship and the most appropriate location of care. From the inception of the welfare state the delivery of care to dependants by women within the home has been a central plank of this particular vision of community care. Beveridge was unashamedly clear in his pronouncement of women's role: '. . . women do vital, though unpaid work, without which their husbands could not do their paid work and without which the nation could not continue' (Beveridge 1942: para 108). Later pronouncements were less straightforwardly honest, but had a similar underlying message:

> Whatever level of public expenditure proves practicable and however it is distributed, the primary sources of support and care for old people are informal and voluntary. These spring from the personalities of kinship, friendship and neighbourhood. They are irreplaceable. It is the role of public authorities to sustain and where necessary, develop – but never to displace – such support and care. Care in the community must mean care by the community.
>
> (DHSS 1981: 3)

Finch and Groves's key observation that '. . . in practice, community care equals care by family and in practice care by family equals care by women' (1980: 494) was, perhaps, the beginning of both a powerfully influential critique of such ideology *and* a persuasive characterization of caring as an oppressive and exhausting burden. At the same time, a developing awareness of new patterns of family life, of prolonged ageing, and of rapidly changing employment patterns raised anxiety about the availability of women and families to care for older, frail dependants. The notion that such changes heralded a decline in family obligations and an overwhelming increase in the 'burden' of aged people in need of care from an ever-decreasing pool of carers has been particularly pervasive.

The twin themes of a critique of women's ascribed role in 'community care' and the anxieties about the sequelae of demographic change have encouraged investigation along a number of lines. First, the characteristics of carers, the identification of their caring activities and their position in 'hierarchies' or 'networks' of care; second, the exploration of the range of experiences associated with caring and the personal costs involved in its delivery; and lastly, the normative bases on which kinship responsibilities and obligations are worked out in practice. While there are clearly overlaps between the three groups of studies, the first two give insights primarily into the way in which care obligations are distributed and the consequences of those patterns of distribution for individual carers, while the third gives some insights into the processes of negotiation and the interpretation of values which result in such characteristic patterns. In spite of these differences in emphasis, all three groups of studies yield data which challenge the attitudinal assumptions of community care policy regarding older people. We review each in turn in the following sections.

Carers and caring: patterns and distribution

The OPCS study of informal carers remains the most comprehensive source of information regarding the identification of carers for older people (Green 1988; OPCS 1992). It was conducted as part of the General Household Survey in 1985, and repeated in 1990. The results show that there were 6.8 million carers in Britain during 1990, of whom 3.9 million were women and 2.9 million were men. Given the larger proportion of women in the general population, these figures seem at first to counter the feminist argument that women are vastly over-represented as carers. However, further examination reveals that women are more likely to take the main responsibility for caring and to devote many more hours to caring activities than men. Further, 34 per cent of single women aged between 45 and 64 years are carers, compared with 21 per cent of single men of the same age (L. Clarke 1995).

These analyses of the OPCS data (L. Clarke 1995) also show that there was an increase of 2 per cent in the numbers of men and women providing informal care to an older person between 1985 and 1990. While co-residence declined slightly due to an increase in the numbers of people looking after their aged parents or parents-in-law within separate households, the greatest majority of caring took place within one home. Carers who were co-resident spent on average 53 hours per week on caring activities, compared to nine hours spent caring by those in another household. Co-resident carers provided more physical and personal care than those who were non-resident – activities which have been shown to be particularly difficult and arduous (Parker 1990). The greatest time given over to caring activities was spent by the spouses of older people, for whom there was no gender difference (L. Clarke 1995). For other relationships, women provided considerably more care than men (Arber and Ginn 1990), with neighbours and friends contributing little to caring activities.

Class differences are visible in the provision of informal care, with working-class men being more likely to deliver the time-consuming and physically arduous co-resident care than middle-class men (Arber and Ginn 1992).

Other studies have rarely highlighted these disparities, although Shanas *et al.* (1968), Abrams (1979, 1980), Taylor and Ford (1983) and Giarchi (1996) have shown that class differentials are a determining factor in the proximity of residence between family members, and that proximity is highly significant in influencing patterns of caring. Giarchi (1996) draws together a number of studies which further suggest that in traditional rural and urban areas, and in areas with high levels of religious affiliation, contact between non-kin is higher. As Giarchi notes, a number of factors seem to contribute to this finding:

> ... the contact between non kin and older people who are lower down the social scale in the rural (and urban areas) ... is more frequent than that between relatives; this is often influenced by proximity and the length and strength of the relationship. The lack of public transport or the use of a car are also additional factors in blocking contact between persons on lower incomes.
>
> (Giarchi 1996: 143)

A long tradition of sociological studies (Townsend 1957; Young and Willmott 1957; Wenger 1984, 1989) shows that household arrangements are plural and diverse, but that within a range of possible types, the family provides the bulk of informal care and support to older people. Further, as Qureshi and Walker (1989) point out on the basis of their study of older people and their families in Sheffield, the primary caring relationship remains between adult daughters and their aged mothers. Qureshi and Walker (1989) identify a clear hierarchy of obligation within family groups which leads to the predominance of this relationship. They describe such a hierarchy as reflecting

> ... a traditional Western normative preference structure. The rules are that close relatives are preferred to more distant ones, any relative is preferred to a non-relative, and female relatives are preferred to male relatives.
>
> (Qureshi and Walker 1989: 123)

The presence of such overwhelming evidence of family-based care delivered primarily by the spouses and daughters of older people has led some authors to conclude that such patterns reflect the existence of particular attitudes within the general population. Phillipson, for example (1993: 51), quotes from Wenger to make this point:

> Research from a wide cross section of developed countries demonstrates that not only does most care come from the family ... but that most people think that this is where the responsibility should lie.
>
> (Wenger 1984: 14)

Such assumptions have been highly influential in framing the 'conceptual map' (Phillipson 1993: 52) of the family life of old people used by investigators. This leads to an almost automatic assumption that reliance on the family is, and will continue to be, at the centre of ideas about caring. As Phillipson notes, '. . . lay, government and some academic views have become stuck in something of a time warp' (1993: 50) of conventional wisdom in which several 'truths' are believed to be self-evident. First, that old people still live near to at least one child; second, that old people who have children see them regularly; and third, that old people who need care want to be cared for by their children. A fourth 'truth' may be added to this list, namely that adult children wish to care for their aged parents.

The evidence from the empirical studies reviewed above suggests that the first two of these 'truths' are under increasing challenge. The proximity of children to their parents may no longer be taken for granted, particularly in middle-class populations and 'non-traditional' rural and urban areas; while intervening factors, such as religion, income, environment, transport, and the proximity and availability of long-term friendships with non-kin may be just as important as kinship in determining patterns of care and support. Perhaps even more significantly, the evidence reviewed above draws attention to the widespread prevalence of older people who are themselves caring for an older spouse. This latter situation, to which comparatively little attention has been paid, is likely to be an ever-increasing scenario bringing with it a new set of questions and problems requiring investigation.

The third and fourth 'truths', regarding the care preferences of older people and their families, have recently been subjected to critical analysis from two sources. First from studies which highlight the negative experiential consequences of caring; and second from studies which examine explicitly attitudes to care, and which explore how these are translated into action.

The experience of caring

A paradoxical observation of studies of the emotional response to care giving is that in spite of very high degrees of mental, physical and financial stress, caregivers are frequently reluctant to accept help, especially if 'help' means admission into institutional care for their relative. For example, Morris et al. (1988) in a review of the caregivers of dementia sufferers found that 40 per cent of their sample were clinically depressed with symptoms of stress running at three times that of the general population. Of these, many expressed guilt at their perceived failure to be the 'ideal' caregiver and found the prospect of institutional care distressing. While it is tempting to assume that such findings merely confirm positive attitudes towards family care, studies are available which suggest a more complex relationship between caregiver strain and reluctance to accept or seek help. Many studies are available which give some insights into this relationship (see for example Equal Opportunities Commission 1981; Lewis and Meredith 1989; Qureshi and Walker 1989; Pollitt *et al.* 1991; Seale and Cartwright 1994); one example will be reviewed here.

Lewis and Meredith (1989), who interviewed 41 women who had cared for their mothers on a co-resident basis, identified a number of issues which compelled daughters to assume exclusive caring roles. First, there was the difficulty of knowing *when* to ask for help. A common experience was that help had to be asked for, rather than being automatically offered at any stage of illness. This made some daughters persevere with daunting caring responsibilities in an attempt to present a 'coping' identity to the outside world. As daughters' mental and physical health became compromised by such long-term strain, their ability to ask for help diminished. Second, social isolation was a common experience particularly during the later stages of caring. This was associated both with daughters' feelings that no one else could care adequately for their mothers' personal needs and with an almost complete lack of knowledge about the availability of help and support. Third, when help was given, daughters reported that it was often inappropriate or inadequate to meet their needs. Lastly, on the occasions when mothers were admitted into institutional care, daughters perceived a 'lack of appreciation' (Lewis and Meredith 1989: 196) on the part of many paid carers of the meaning of caring for the daughters themselves. Staff were perceived as 'taking over' from daughters, leading to a lack of self-worth and a sense of exclusion at a stressful time of transition. Here, the positive aspects of caring, which had coexisted with the more negative features, were suddenly withdrawn. In particular, the intimacy which had developed between mother and daughter over a long period of time was interrupted sharply, and there were little or no opportunities made available for its reinstatement.

These findings suggest that attitudes to caring have to be explored in relation to the particular circumstances in which it is conducted. Assuming that a reluctance to ask for help is evidence of a strongly positive attitude towards family care has been shown by researchers such as Lewis and Meredith to be untenable, misleading, and requiring further detailed investigation.

Attitudes and actions regarding the provision and receipt of care

Evidence has recently become available from studies which suggest that, while family ties remain strong, the family is not necessarily seen as the most appropriate source of help and support for older people. Older people themselves seem to prefer to maintain their independence, while younger people do not automatically see themselves as the 'first port of call' for assistance with ageing parents. A few studies have explored the ways in which beliefs and attitudes about family obligations are translated into

practice, suggesting that obligations are not fixed, but that they are negotiated according to family circumstances and with due attention to maintaining a balance between dependence and reciprocity.

Finch and Mason (1990, 1993) conducted a study in the Greater Manchester area during 1985, collecting both quantitative and qualitative data
about family obligations and attitudes to providing support of all types.
Their results suggest that, while people generally see it as appropriate that
adult children do 'something' to support their parents, there is little broad
agreement as to exactly what form that support should take. Finch and
Mason concluded that, while perceived obligations were fulfilled in radically different ways according to the histories of family relationships and
other unique circumstances, certain principles were followed and preserved.
These principles were derived from commitments between individual children and parents that had developed over the years of their relationship.
Commitments involved a process of long-term reciprocity:

> ... accepting help – and then giving something in return – is the engine
> which drives the process of developing commitments ... reciprocal
> help is a crucial factor in understanding how family relationships
> operate. It means that each child will build a set of commitments with
> her parents which is different from each of her brothers' and sisters'
> commitments. When people talk about responsibilities to their relatives
> they mean responsibilities arrived at in this way ... not obligations
> which flow simply from the genealogical link.
>
> (Finch 1995: 54)

Finch and Mason's findings are reflected in Donald and Gordon's (1991)
study of informal care and older people in Scotland and in the results of a
study by Salvage et al. (1989) in Wales. More broadly, national opinion
surveys such as the British Social Attitudes Survey (McGlone et al. 1996)
and the Eurobarometer surveys of public attitudes to older people and
ageing (Walker 1993) show patterns of response that could be interpreted
using Finch and Mason's (1993) concepts of individual commitments and
long-term reciprocity.

Several hypotheses may be developed on the basis of these findings (Finch
1995). First, family responsibilities may be regarded as fluid and variable,
rather than fixed, by large numbers of the population. Second, problems of
role conflict between the demands of caring, employment and other pressures may be differentially interpreted and resolved. Third, achieving a balance between dependence and reciprocity may be considered to be critically
important by both older people and their families. Lastly, 'reciprocity'
and 'dependence' will have a range of meanings depending upon negotia-
tions within specific interpersonal relationships. Each of these will have
relevance to the ways in which the care of dying relatives is perceived and
undertaken.

Bereavement, grief and mourning

Bereavement is a virtually universal experience. At some point in our lives we will almost all lose through death family members, friends or colleagues. As we get older, such losses are likely to be a repeated feature of life, and we will mark them in a culturally determined and socially sanctioned manner by attendance at a funeral or other mourning ceremony. Some bereavements may engender powerful feelings of grief, in which sadness and suffering encircle those who were particularly close to the dead person. For some, grief is never fully eradicated and becomes a central part of everyday life. For others, grief is more transitory and has less impact on daily life. Littlewood (1992: 40–59) gives a detailed account of the range of emotions which may be experienced during bereavement, giving some sense of their sheer unpredictability and paradoxicality. The experience of bereavement will be influenced by a range of factors, including the nature of the bereaved individual's relationship with the dead person; the manner and timing of the death; the degree to which death is expected or unexpected; and the age and 'social worth' of the dead person. A 1998 television documentary about the parents of children who were killed in the Aberfan disaster which had occurred some 30 years earlier bears witness to the enduring power of grief in some circumstances. The film revealed, in a vivid and moving way, how the parents' sense of cataclysmic loss has never diminished, only become more bearable as time has passed. Further, their individually experienced loss has, to some extent, been shared by the whole local community and the wider country. Media coverage of the disaster evoked an acute, if transitory, sense of grief among people who had probably never heard of Aberfan previously, let alone had any personal contact with its inhabitants. More recently the tragic events at Dunblane and the extraordinary scenes associated with the death of Diana, Princess of Wales, have reminded us of the commonality of grief and the interface between its individual and social manifestations. In all of these examples, personal grief intertwined with public ritual and the impromptu communal expression of sadness.

How may we make sense of this interweaving of the personal and private with the interpersonal and public? An examination of the ways in which bereavement, grief and mourning have been conceptualized may shed some light on the complexity of the relationship.

Let us start by clarifying the accepted definitions of bereavement, grief and mourning. We show here some definitions put forward by Wendell-Moller (1996: 108–9):

• Bereavement is an essential component of grief. Literally speaking, to be bereaved means to be deprived, to have something taken away . . . bereavement can be defined as the sense of deprivation or loss generated by the loss of another person.

- Grief is an intense emotional response to bereavement that involves sorrow and suffering . . . bereavement precedes grief but is not necessarily followed by it.
- Mourning is the behavioural expression of the emotional anguish of grief but may not always reflect inner feelings.

Wendell-Moller (1996) argues that the behavioural and emotional manifestations of bereavement are socially determined or constructed and, as such, are historically and culturally specific. For example, each society or cultural grouping within that society will have its own particular ways of fashioning mourning rituals, or 'rites of passage'. These rituals will reflect the predominant forms of belief that are held and will express communally the fundamental changes and transitions believed to be associated with death. The transitions associated with the change in status from 'parent' to 'bereaved parent', or from 'wife' to 'widow' are clear examples of the types of social transition involved here, while for those with religious beliefs, the transition of the deceased from a corporeal to a spiritual form will be of critical importance. Beyond these communal rituals, members of each society will demonstrate particular patterns of behaviour towards those who have been bereaved. In our Western culture avoidance and voyeurism have been identified as two common, albeit deeply unhelpful, patterns of behaviour which we tend to exhibit towards bereaved people (Littlewood 1992). Some authors have linked the apparent decline of religiously inspired mourning rituals and patterns of social avoidance in contemporary Western society to a lengthening and deepening of the individual course of grief (Gorer 1965; Ariès 1976). Lofland (1985: 180–1) argues that in Western culture bereavement is experienced as particularly intense and tragic, and that a number of circumstances have combined to reproduce this intensity. These all place special emphasis on the importance of individuality and the material world, and encourage a world-view in which death is regarded as the ultimate form of loss. The conditions Lofland identifies are:

1 a relational pattern which links individuals to a small number of highly significant others;
2 a definition of death as personal annihilation and as unusual and tragic except among the aged;
3 selves who take very seriously their emotional states; and
4 interactional settings which provide rich opportunities to contemplate loss.

Personal experiences of grief are clearly influenced by, and must be interpreted within, a cultural and social context. This insight is perhaps the key to understanding the links between personal experiences of bereavement and their resonance at the wider social and societal levels. In the West, bereavement has been studied extensively and has been subject to a variety of theoretical constructions during the twentieth century. All of these take the individual as the basic unit of analysis and in so doing have focused attention even more closely on the *individual* manifestations of grief, and the process of *individual adjustment* to bereavement. While these constructions take the form of 'ideal types' rather than attempts to capture the full range of human experience in an empirically accurate way, many of them have infiltrated the public and professional consciousness. In so doing they have had a powerful influence on the ways in which we make sense of grief and loss. It might be argued, following Lofland (1985), that bereavement models have become frameworks of social meaning within which we try to 'fit' and make sense of feelings experienced at an individual level.

Many texts are available which offer detailed accounts of the origins and formulations of the various theorizations of bereavement (Stroebe and Stroebe 1987; Littlewood 1992; Walter 1994). Here, our aim is to draw on these texts to give a brief sketch of the key themes of three influential models. We will then turn to an examination of some sociological and social–psychological critiques of these models which have emerged recently. For ease of reference, we set them out in schematic form.

The illness and disease model: a biological explanation

- Based on the early work of Lindemann (1944) and Engel (1961, 1962).
- Sees grief as a 'sickness': a form of disease.
- Regards grief as a syndrome with predictable symptoms and course.
- Views grief as a biological stressor giving rise to a range of physiological responses: depression; anxiety; physical illness.
- Classifies some forms of grief as 'morbid' or 'abnormal'.

The psycho-dynamic model: an intra-psychic explanation

- Based on the early work of Freud (1917) and Klein (1948); subsequently developed by Pincus (1976).
- Concerned with the intra-psychic 'world'.
- Concerned with the threat of grief to intra-psychic stability.
- Identifies grief as a form of severe depression.
- Conceptualizes grief as slow, painful and ambivalent: involving a tension between separation and attachment.
- Sees grief as having a particular purpose: a recognition of loss and emotional detachment from the dead person.

The attachment–disengagement model: a reconstitutive explanation

- Based on Bowlby's analysis (1980) of the mother–child relationship.
- Utilizes a theory of attachment which hypothesizes that all emotionally significant relationships are characterized by instinctive patterns of response which reflect the mother–child nexus.

- Sees death or separation provoking a range of responses which mirror those elicited in children deprived of their mother-figure: anger, weeping, despair, searching behaviours.
- Sees this phase of 'behavioural disorganization' eventually giving way to 'reorganization', marked by a relocation of affective bonds to others.
- Contributes to formulations of grief as a psycho-social transition (Murray Parkes 1970; Raphael 1984), as a collection of stages (Kübler-Ross 1969) or tasks (Worden 1982).

As Walter points out, there are extensive areas of common ground among these theoretical models. As a result the sophisticated analyses with which they are underpinned are often distilled in practice by virtue of a 'selective reading' (1996: 8) to one or two essential messages. These readings, Walter argues, emphasize detachment from the dead and de-emphasize the possibility of their continued presence in our social and individual lives. They reflect the secular and individualistic culture of late twentieth-century society, and in particular our concern with the 'healthy' functioning of the autonomous individual:

> This body of work has been widely read to say that the purpose of grief is the reconstitution of an autonomous individual who can in large measure leave the deceased behind and form new attachments. The process by which this is believed to be achieved is the working through and resolution of feelings – the psychological literature on grief is full of discussion of anger, guilt, depression, sadness and a whole range of feelings with which bereaved people may have to come to terms. These concepts of the purpose and process of grief form much of the conventional wisdom . . . of bereavement counselling.
>
> (Walter 1996: 7)

Further, popular conceptions of bereavement tend to focus on personal adaptations to, and recovery from, the 'sickness' of grief. They have tapped into wider preoccupations with medical and psycho-therapeutic explanations of suffering and in so doing have encouraged the representation of grief as either 'normal' or 'abnormal'. Concern has focused on the identification of, first, factors which prompt 'abnormal' grieving; second, patterns of behaviour or 'symptoms' which signify 'abnormal' grieving; and third, the development of interventions to aid the resolution of 'abnormal' grief. Grief and bereavement counselling have thus assumed a special importance as a means of relocating bereaved individuals on the path of 'normal' grieving and facilitating their detachment from the dead person.

Emergent critiques draw attention to the ways in which the complexity, variation and social nature of grief as a human experience have been fundamentally undermined by these widely accepted formulations of bereavement. Walter (1996) suggests, for example, that 'detachment' is not necessarily seen as a goal of grieving by those who have been bereaved. Rather a central aim may be the 'reconstruction' of the biography of their relationship with the dead person by means of conversation with others who have known that person. Through this restitutive process attachment to the deceased is strengthened and given meaning within the ongoing life of the survivor. It becomes part of a refashioned sense of self-identity. Walter draws on his own personal experience and on the theoretical writings of Giddens (1991) about identity formation in late modern society to make this claim. Walter's analysis might be criticized for assuming that all bereaved people have others with whom to share recollections of the dead person. Clearly, in some circumstances this may not be possible. Those who have experienced neo-natal death; death of a spouse following a life of moderate social isolation; or death in circumstances such as suicide may not have an opportunity to gather with others to make sense of death and to reconstruct the biography of their dead companion.

Research by Rees (1997) suggests that conversation is not the only means of continuing attachment to the dead that may be sought by bereaved people. Rees bases his analysis on research among bereaved spouses conducted in mid-Wales and explores in some detail experiences of those who claim to have continued spiritual contact with their dead partner. Rather than assuming that such experiences are evidence of pathological grief, Rees suggests that they are part of the usual experience of grief for many. However, fear of mockery or of disbelief makes it difficult for bereaved people to express themselves in their own terms. For some bereaved people belief in a spiritual dimension may coexist with material existence: this is not, however, part of the philosophy which underpins the traditional bereavement models:

> ... the bereaved are deprived of their own interpretation of what is happening ... the psychological theory also carries the implication that if the bereaved have hallucinations of the dead they have not completed the mourning process and, in that sense, are still emotionally disabled. It does not accept the possibility that the widowed may have been enlarged by the experience and their lives therefore enhanced. A spiritual explanation opens up a new perspective for the bereaved as it implies a continued existence after death which, though it cannot be proved, is affirmed by the near presence of the deceased.
>
> (Rees 1997: 203)

The importance, for many bereaved people, of continuing contact with those who have died, and the belief in a spiritual dimension highlighted by Rees and by Walter, exposes a neglect of the sheer variety of experiences and beliefs associated with bereavement. The central role ethnicity plays in the conceptualization of bereavement may be particularly underestimated in the schemata developed by Western bereavement theorists. For example,

Rees examines attitudes to bereavement in Japan, showing the central role of dead 'ancestors' in Japanese life. The ancestors become important sources of ongoing support and inspiration with whom to share the tribulations and triumphs of the material life:

> Japanese culture encourages the living to maintain a relationship with the dead and the continuance of the relationship is facilitated by the presence of the family shrine . . . The family altar is used as though it is a 'hot line'. The living can light incense and symbolically make a telephone call to discuss current problems with a loved and cherished ancestor, the *kami* of the shrine. When happy they can smile and share their good feelings with him; if sad they can shed tears in his presence. The ancestors can be cherished, fed, berated and idealised by all the family members. By this means the living maintain a continuous relationship with those they have loved and lost.
>
> (Rees 1997: 30)

Gender is also coming to light as a significant contributor to patterns of grieving and to ways of making sense of loss. For example, Stroebe (1996) found that men use coping strategies during bereavement that are very different from those employed by women. Similarly, Riches and Dawson (1997) found during research with bereaved parents that fathers and mothers tended to orient themselves to grief in different ways, and have to negotiate jointly a shared meaning of loss through their marital relationship.

In late modern society 'talk' and conversation, either with others, with the dead person, or inwardly, may be the primary means by which grief and loss are assuaged and the special place and identity of the dead person negotiated and reaffirmed. Overarching religious narratives emphasizing the importance of an afterlife and the worthiness of the dead person for immortality have, for many, been replaced by an almost celebratory emphasis on events or critical moments during the process of dying or the life of the dead person (Seale 1995). For others, religious rituals retain their importance as a means of containing and making sense of loss. Bereavement, grief and mourning in this sense become continuations and reflections of the rich variety of social, cultural and interpersonal life, rather than experiences which can be explained neatly by reference to a particular theoretical model.

We begin to see then that processes of ageing, of caring and of grieving may be closely intertwined in the lives of many individuals in late modern culture. As we grow older we may experience multiple minor losses in our individual capacities and abilities. In so doing we may become increasingly dependent upon a significant other, usually a spouse; that person in turn may be facing similar problems associated with ageing and the advancement of chronic illness. In later life we are also likely to experience multiple bereavements resulting from the deaths of our peers. By such means the worlds of the living and of the dead are brought closer together. Increasingly, social commentators are beginning to recognize that all these aspects of 'living with dying' are important elements of human experience. The normative separation of life from death, encouraged by earlier theories of bereavement, has been called into question and we are encountering a greater willingness to emphasize the continuities between the world of the survivor and the memory of the dead person. Such discourses move us towards a new construction of ageing, dying and grieving in late modernity, and beyond crude formulations of these as forms of 'taboo' in contemporary culture. In such circumstances it also becomes more possible to talk of ethical considerations surrounding care at the end of life.

3 The ethics of dying

It can prove difficult to keep up with the sheer volume of current writing and commentary on euthanasia, and related topics. In several countries, most notably the United States, the Netherlands and Australia, these have become major areas of public debate and discussion, going well beyond the technical considerations of medicine, ethics and the law. One of the reasons for this growing public interest in issues of end-of-life care must be seen to lie in the pervasive sense of doubt and mistrust which characterizes late modern culture. This has led to a profound scepticism about the benefits of medicine's ability to extend life, coupled with an increasingly articulated unease about the power of professionals to control end-of-life decision making. As the debate rages, the sectional voices of a variety of interest groups become louder and the focus of argument can appear increasingly specialized. So it is important to gain a perspective on the subject which takes a longer and more comparative view. Historical and sociological writings (particularly the latter) on euthanasia are not extensive but they do offer us an opportunity to view the issues in their wider context, and not to become focused unduly on isolated areas of the field.

For these reasons we shall try in this chapter to explain why it might be that euthanasia and its correlates became important in the closing decades of the twentieth century. Opportunities will also be sought to draw on empirical studies from differing countries in order to understand how public attitudes and professional practices may be relating to one another. Above all, however, the chapter will emphasize the point made by Howarth and Jefferys, that 'the current debate on euthanasia is at least partly about agency, about who does and who should control the decisions to hasten or procure death' (1996: 381). To focus on agency in this way provides some opportunity for understanding how individual, social and societal issues

Figure 3.1 The terminology of euthanasia

Euthanasia	From the Greek *euthanatos*, meaning 'good death' in the sense of dying painlessly or easily. Now more typically used to refer to a deliberate intervention or omission intended to end life in order to relieve intractable suffering. *Euthanatos* needs to be distinguished from another Greek term, *Kalos Thanatos* meaning 'good death' in the sense of dying in an ideal way, according to a set of culturally sanctioned behaviours.
Voluntary (or active) euthanasia	Any action or omission that ends intentionally the life of someone else, on the request of that person.
Involuntary (or passive) euthanasia	Conduct designed to end the life of someone who desires to go on living.
Non-voluntary euthanasia	Conduct designed to end the life of someone who has never expressed any wish to die or survive, and who cannot currently communicate.
Slow euthanasia	The clinical practice of treating a terminally ill patient in a manner that will assuredly lead to a comfortable death, but not too quickly.
Physician-assisted suicide	When a doctor provides assistance to bring about a death, but the patient performs the final and necessary act.
Double effect	Actions intended to relieve suffering, but which may also hasten death.
Withdrawal of treatment	When a decision is reached that it would not be in the interests of the patient to continue life-prolonging treatment, though attention to comfort is sustained.
Withholding treatment	When a decision is taken, in the interests of the patient, not to embark upon life-prolonging treatment.
Advance directive (living will)	A document drawn up by a patient who is mentally competent, to indicate views on particular treatments at a later stage.
Slippery slope	The idea that the legalization of euthanasia, however circumscribed, will lead inevitably to its wider adoption in other contexts.

may combine to produce the complex 'problem' of euthanasia which is confronting late modern societies and which is having an important impact on thinking relating to palliative care.

One measure of the extent to which a social issue is the subject of tensions and dissensions in society is the degree to which it is surrounded by debates about definition and disagreements over terminology. This chapter will in no sense seek to resolve these, indeed such clarity may be neither possible nor desirable. Figure 3.1 does, however, give a basic summary of some of the terms to be found in the debate and can be referred to as a guide to reading.

Euthanasia: historical and social perspectives

The foundation of contemporary medical ethics on death and dying originates in the societies of classical Greece and Rome. For example, Cowley *et al.* (1992) show that the medical literature of these times evinces a selfless concern for the health and well-being of the patient, coupled with a reticence on the part of physicians to attempt futile treatment for serious and painful afflictions, in which the Hippocratic injunction called upon them to 'at least do no harm'. Indeed the Hippocratic tests imply that one function of prognostication was to protect physicians from taking responsibility for unmanageable or terminal patients. Herein lies the origin of the idea that death constitutes a failure for medicine.

In medieval Europe, however, it was the priest rather than the physicians who brought comfort as death approached and Christianity influenced deeply the practice of a medicine wherein the sanctity of life was paramount. With the Renaissance, the authority of medical thinking expanded and alongside came ambitions to prolong life and establish a scientific basis to medical practice. The conditions were now in place for an increasingly secularized medicine in which positivist thinking portrayed death as the enemy of life. Pappas (1996) argues, however, that in the twentieth century the rise in chronic, degenerative conditions has fuelled the beginnings of a modern medical euthanasia controversy. Whilst huge progress has been made to curb epidemics of infectious disease, new problems arise in ageing populations with high levels of cardio-vascular, cerebro-vascular and other long-term illnesses. In turn we have come to see the limits, indeed the nemesis of medicine (Illich 1976), generated from within by the profession's own quest for influence and power. It has been accompanied by an increasing interest in and concern about medical euthanasia on the part of health professionals.

There has also, of course, been growing *public* interest in the matter, and organizations concerned to promote the case for euthanasia were formed in Britain in 1935 and three years later in the USA. Williams (1992) contends that the emergence of cancer as a perceived source of painful and grim death was responsible for these developments, but he also notes that in Britain in the intervening years the euthanasia movement has failed consistently in its paramount aim. The first euthanasia bill was debated in the British parliament in 1936 yet there has still been no change in the law. By contrast, Williams points out, the modern hospice movement which did not get underway until some 30 years later has made huge strides in service development, professional practice and education. Supporters of the modern hospices have of course been particularly opposed to euthanasia and from the outset have lobbied against it.

In another paper Williams (1989) shows the way in which, on the evidence of opinion polls, public attitudes to euthanasia seem to have differed in Britain and the United States. In Britain public opinion from the 1930s appears strongly in favour of statements permitting doctors deliberately to take life. Such attitudes are not in evidence in the United States until the 1970s, and even then are somewhat equivocal. By contrast, the acceptance of ideas of open communication about and awareness of a terminal condition arrives earlier in the United States than in Britain and seems to be more strongly held. Williams suggests that the wish to have full information about both diagnosis and prognosis in terminal illness was not general or clear-cut in Britain or America in the 1950s; but that a radical change towards this preference has occurred in America during the 1960s and 1970s, while in Britain the change remains 'cautious and somewhat ambiguous' (1989: 204). He also points out that part of the basis of the voluntary euthanasia movement in Britain in the 1930s was a reaction against medical heroism and what were perceived as futile, unnecessary efforts to prolong life. In the United States this reaction was not to come until much later, in the context of a society which for most of the twentieth century placed enormous collective faith in the ability of modern medicine to triumph even over the threat of mortal illness.

Two American sociologists, Caddell and Newton (1995), report on five surveys of public opinion toward euthanasia and the physician's role in performing it. The surveys were conducted in the United States between 1977 and 1988 and involved a total of 8834 respondents. Over the decade an average of 62 per cent of the sample found active euthanasia acceptable and almost 45 per cent considered that suicide was acceptable in a terminally ill patient. These attitudes became more prevalent as the decade advanced. The data showed that Americans tend to draw a distinction between the suicide of a terminally ill person and active euthanasia under the care of a physician, with a preference for the doctor to perform this role in the dying process. Those who favour euthanasia and physician-assisted suicide tend to be less religious and more highly educated. In addition to those with no professed religion, Jews and liberal Protestants also hold views strongly in favour. Conservative Protestants were found to be least supportive, but even among this group 54 per cent endorsed active euthanasia and 33 per cent considered the suicide of a terminally ill person to be acceptable. The figures for Catholics were 63 per cent and 43 per cent, respectively.

Caddell and Newton point out that the importance of religion in determining American attitudes to these subjects is not surprising. Although public institutions in the United States are largely secularized, religious worldviews and associations remain important. They describe a 'restructuring' process, in both politics and religion, in which the landscape has become increasingly polarized into 'conservative' and 'liberal' camps (1995: 1679). Given the marked decline in political and religious liberalism in the period since the surveys they report were conducted, the authors speculate on the impact this may have on public opinion towards euthanasia and related issues.

Nicholas Christakis, a sociologist and a physician, has examined why such attitudes might be prevalent within American society and how in particular they relate to modern medical practice. He argues that:

> As a result of both the proliferation of medical technology and the sequestration of large numbers of dying patients in institutions, contemporary American physicians, more so than ever before, influence the timing, rapidity, and painlessness of patients' deaths.
>
> (Christakis 1996: 15)

In this context, euthanasia might be seen as almost a logical extension of the physician's role in managing death. By these means, euthanasia achieves a new legitimacy, fuelled in part by the very paradox that modern medicine often increases suffering when it prolongs life. The professional concerns of doctors on such matters also occur in the context of critical scrutiny of financial allocation within health care systems and the assertion that futile attempts to prolong life represent a waste of finite resources.

This can mean that decisions relating to the withholding or withdrawal of treatment become a regular feature of clinical practice, particularly in specialties like intensive care. In these settings formal medical decisions to limit treatment or not to resuscitate critically ill patients frequently precede death (Koch et al. 1994; Simpson 1994; Searle 1996). The trend is also in evidence in other areas of medicine (Faber-Langendoen 1992; Pijnenborg et al. 1995). At the heart of this is the recognition that such decisions are *sequential* in character, rather than single events. Accordingly, attention has focused on the distinction between 'killing' and 'letting die' (Rachels 1975; Cartwright 1996), with practice often seeking to eliminate any 'proximate relationship' (Hoyt 1995) or causative link in a chain of actions and inactions on the part of health professionals, which eventually results in the death of the patient.

Medicine's dominion over end-of-life decision making, a strong emphasis on matters of individual autonomy and consumerism in health care, coupled with increasing constraints on resource allocation, have all combined to promote debate about euthanasia. The implications are far-reaching and range from the individual circumstances of patients described as being in a persistent vegetative state, to very wide questions of policy and demography. The slippery slope argument against euthanasia, for example, is predicated on the notion that legalization could allow for the mass disposal of groups deemed non-viable, costly to support or otherwise dispensable. In the palliative care context discussion has centred much more around whether the means to relieve suffering are available to medicine and the impact this has on requests for euthanasia. Precisely how such a request is constituted, however, is itself problematic and calls for some detailed consideration.

Euthanasia: requests and responses

Against this shifting background of public debate and legal change, there has been increasing interest on the part of researchers in identifying empirical evidence about requests for euthanasia, together with the resulting responses. To date most of this work tends to focus on the experience of professionals (mainly doctors) and looks at the frequency with which such requests occur, together with the responses which are made and the general predisposition of professionals to the euthanasia question. Some work has tried to develop an understanding from the perspective of patients and also from informal carers. Before considering such data, however, it is important to interject a note of sociological caution. Three points are worthy of comment.

First, 'requests for euthanasia' should not be read off as unproblematic utterances, subject to purely rational debate. Although euthanasia movements are located within a rationalist tradition, it is a characteristic of the subject matter that debates surrounding it may have to acknowledge the limits of modern, scientific rationality. Second, 'requests for euthanasia' must be seen as complex *social constructions*; they are therefore only to be understood within the context in which they occur. What constitutes a 'request for euthanasia' may vary between the settings of hospital, home or hospice. Such a 'request' may be heard differently by individual members of the health care team, and certainly the response will vary accordingly. Doctors for example may receive more *direct* requests, because they are perceived as having the wherewithal (though not necessarily the will) to act on them; nurses by contrast may encounter more *indirect* requests, in a context where deliberate killing may conflict with the nursing ethos of care. Third, and this is most important, 'requests for euthanasia' should be seen as ideological constructs, insofar as they may be used to promote or challenge particular viewpoints and value positions. As presented in the research and professional literature and as examined in more public debates, such evidence serves purposes beyond mere description. So when making sense of evidence or arguments on the subject we do well to foster a sociological scepticism rooted in such questions as: who is presenting this data; how was it gathered; for what purpose; and to favour what ends?

Various recent studies report on the extent to which doctors, in several different countries, have been asked by patients to hasten their death. The tendency for this varies, but in affluent countries is reported at fairly high levels. In the United Kingdom, Ward and Tate (1994) report that 60 per cent of the doctors they surveyed had been asked to hasten a patient's death and 12 per cent had taken active steps to do so. In the Netherlands, where euthanasia has been decriminalized, 54 per cent of physicians have acknowledged assisting in at least one death at the patient's request (van der Maas *et al*. 1991) and requests for euthanasia have been experienced by three-quarters of all doctors. Stevens and Hassan (1994) report that 47 per cent of Australian doctors studied had received requests from patients to hasten their deaths and 19 per cent had taken active steps which had brought about the death of a patient. In the USA 50 per cent of oncologists had received requests for euthanasia, with 1.8 per cent complying with euthanasia and 13.5 per cent with physician-assisted suicide (Emmanuel *et al*. 1996). There have been fewer studies of nurses in this context, but Asch (1996) in a study of critical care nurses found a rather low figure in contrast to those for doctors, of 17 per cent who had received requests for euthanasia and 16 per cent who have engaged in the practice; in this study it was also found that 4 per cent of the nurses had hastened a patient's death by merely pretending to provide life-sustaining treatment ordered by a physician.

The study by Emmanuel and colleagues is interesting in that it compared the views of oncologists, patients and the general public. The latter two groups were three times more likely than the oncologists to agree with euthanasia for unremitting pain and functional debility and six times more likely in the case of burden on the family and where life was viewed as meaningless (Emmanuel *et al*. 1996). Such studies, which present hypothetical vignettes to their subjects, differ from those which report patients' personal views about their situation or actions which they have themselves taken. A few examples of such studies now exist, and these emanate from the context of specialist palliative care services, so must be viewed in that light.

For example, Harvey Chochinov and colleagues (1995) found that in a sample of 200 patients being cared for in two hospital palliative care units in Manitoba, Canada, 44 per cent acknowledged at least a fleeting desire for death, but this was often brief and not sustained. However 8.5 per cent of the sample did appear to have a more sustained desire for death and over a half of these were rated as depressed. At the Daw House Hospice in Adelaide, Australia, Hunt and colleagues (1995) report that over a two-year

Figure 3.2   The wish to die earlier and requests for euthanasia

---

- Looking back now and taking (the deceased's) illness into account, do you think that s/he died at the best time – or would it have been better if s/he had died earlier or later?

    Died earlier: 28%

- What about (the deceased)? Did s/he ever say that they wanted to die sooner?

    Die sooner: 24%

- (If yes) did s/he ever say that s/he wanted euthanasia?

    Wanted euthanasia: 3.6%

Source: Seale and Addington-Hall 1997

period 6 per cent of patients had asked 'could you hurry it up?' and a further 6 per cent had said 'please do something now'. Again, it was considered that requests for such interventions are largely tentative and indirect and the authors make the point:

> . . . as suffering is brought under control, positive exchanges encouraged, and loving relationships engendered in a supportive hospice environment, the desire for a quick exit is likely to decrease.
>
> (Hunt *et al.* 1995: 168)

It is this assertion, which has been such a fundamental aspect of hospice philosophy, that is challenged by empirical evidence produced by Seale and Addington-Hall (1994, 1995). The study focuses on a sample of 3696 people dying in 1990 in 20 health authorities in England. Data were gathered by means of structured interviews in the community with people who best knew the circumstances of the deceased person's last year of life; over 80 per cent of interviews were with relatives, and the interviews took place some nine months after the death had occurred. In the course of a long and detailed interview, three key questions were asked relating to wishing to die sooner and euthanasia (Figure 3.2). Responses to these show that over a quarter of respondents said that it would have been better if the person had died earlier; just under a quarter of those who died were reported as having said that they wished to die sooner; and 3.6 per cent of the people who had died were reported to have asked for euthanasia.

So here are some important data, from a representative and population-based sample, rather than a sample of convenience drawn from within a particular clinical service, on the frequency with which people express the wish to die earlier, or request euthanasia. It is what Seale and Addington-Hall show about this 3.6 per cent however that is of most interest. First, it was found that pain was only weakly associated with views about an earlier death, as expressed by respondents and as reported by the dying people themselves; it was however a more significant factor for those with cancer than for those with other conditions. Of those who died from non-malignant causes, *dependency* was the strongest factor associated with the wish to die earlier in the view of respondents; and as reported by the deceased, loss of *control* figured the most strongly. Contrary to the evidence found in public opinion surveys which seek to measure attitudes towards euthanasia, social class, place of residence of the deceased and strength and type of religious faith were found to be largely insignificant in influencing feelings about an earlier death and requests for euthanasia.

Most striking of all, however, were the study findings relating to the role of hospice care in influencing attitudes to an earlier death or euthanasia. It might be hypothesized that those receiving care in hospice would be less likely to request euthanasia. In fact the reverse was found to be the case. Seale and Addington-Hall show, when restricting the analysis to cancer patients, who constitute the vast majority of patients in hospices in the UK, that spending time in a hospice in the last year of life increases the likelihood of a request for euthanasia. The authors found that among cancer patients who had received no hospice care, 3.6 per cent were said to have asked for euthanasia; this compared to 8.8 per cent of those who had received in-patient hospice care during the last year of life. Moreover people who received hospice care were if anything more likely to have respondents who felt it would have been better if they had died earlier, this being 1.7 times more likely than for those who did not receive hospice care.

We have, then, a counter-intuitive finding. Of course, an obvious problem is posed by the time order of events. Did the request for euthanasia precede admission to hospice care or follow it? Similarly, did those who received hospice care have the most complex problems? And could the hospices be expected to compensate for poor care which may have been given elsewhere, thus contributing to a desire for an earlier death or euthanasia? In a further paper Seale *et al.* (1997) offer some commentary. They suggest that the issue is related to the presence of an open awareness context. People in the study who were said to have died in an open awareness context were considerably more likely to say that they wished to die sooner and also to have wanted euthanasia. They were also more likely to have been a hospice in-patient during their last year of life. So paradoxically, there appears to be an elective affinity between the open awareness context which hospice practice may seek to foster and rather positive attitudes towards an earlier death or the possibility of life being ended through euthanasia. These are of course data from only one study, and as the authors acknowledge, they do present certain problems, but nevertheless the careful analysis which has resulted raises interesting questions, both for practitioners and for further research enquiry.

We keep returning therefore to the trajectory of dying in late modern culture and to the emphasis on control over the dying process, particularly through active medical intervention. The manner and timing of death has thus become subject to a range of clinical 'choices' and 'options'. It is apparent from the foregoing discussion that, despite worldwide interest in the questions of euthanasia and physician-assisted suicide, the current state of medical ethics remains contested and confused. We have seen that attempts have been made over time to measure the climate of public opinion on these matters. In Britain these appear to reveal a growing trend of support for the legalization of euthanasia, albeit within the clearly defined circumstances of irreversible coma or very severe pain in a terminal condition. There is however some evidence that there may be a difference between what individuals would choose for themselves and their views as expressed in relation to a fictitious, vignette-like scenario. Studies which focus on older people already facing serious illness and dependency tend to show less positive attitudes to euthanasia than might be predicted by large-scale surveys (High 1993; Kelner 1995; Cicirelli 1997). Donnison and Bryson (1996) agree however that it is age associated with greater religiosity, rather than age alone, which contributes to negative attitudes about euthanasia. The same authors also show that, where the circumstances of euthanasia are carefully defined, then the range of opinions about its social and moral value will be much more widely spread.

The research on advance directives and their use in aiding surrogate decision making has particularly highlighted the circumstantial and dynamic nature of 'public opinion' and it has been reported as an issue in the administration of the Oregon experiment concerning health care rationing in the USA (Bowling 1992). In a different context West (1984) has shown clearly that idealized choices and attitudes about care arrangements may not be related to the *actual* decisions that individuals make, or are constrained to make. Indeed, individuals seem to be confronted with 'a set of overlapping value systems within which specific needs and interests are resolved' (West 1984: 443). The contextual constraints of everyday life and reflexive experience therefore appear to encourage individuals to make and re-make opinions in a dynamic, circumstantial manner, with *general* attitudes becoming a resource pool rather than an exclusive determinant of action. Corr (1993) notes similarly that life experience and attitudes are tightly interrelated and may have a dialectical influence upon each other:

Encounters and attitudes are not independent components of human experience . . . as individuals live out their lives, encounters and attitudes intertwine and interact as the warp and weft of death related experiences. Different types of death related experiences are likely to engender different sorts of attitudes, just as differing attitudes are likely to encourage or to inhibit death related encounters.

(Corr 1993: 28)

The differences between the abstract expression of 'general' opinion and the 'concrete' choices that an individual would make when actually faced with a life-threatening illness may, in part, be an expression of the paradoxical relationship that medicine has established with its public. It may well be that there is anxiety about medical rationing being applied covertly to certain marginal groups in society – the very old, or disabled people, for example, albeit disguised within rhetorics of self-determination, choice and 'the patient's best interests'. The cultural coexistence and cross-cutting impact of ideas about the 'right to die' and the 'right to life' movements bear witness to the current state of flux and what appears to be a 'confused vortex of complementary and opposing trends . . . and a complexity of meanings that are still little explored' (Williams 1989: 208).

In such a context there appears to be no great likelihood of any public consensus on end-of-life care ethics, particularly relating to euthanasia. Instead we see a shifting mosaic within which there is uncertainty and a lack of constancy. Within such a context the activities of Dr Jack Kevorkian can be promulgated; physician-assisted death can be briefly legalized and then recriminalized in the Australian Northern Territory; and in Holland it can become a decriminalized commonplace of medical practice. In Britain, individual 'right to die' cases regularly receive widespread coverage in the press, often followed by counter-arguments from within the hospice movement. It seems likely that such ethical debates concerning end-of-life care will continue. Our hope is that they will become better informed by an appreciation of the historical and cultural determinants of ethical thinking and practice and by the increased understanding and tolerance which such an appreciation may bring.

PART II

The philosophy and practice of palliative care

Introduction to Part II

In Part II we move from the wider social context to concentrate on a more detailed discussion of the philosophy and practice of palliative care. We have made a particular effort to locate this discussion within a *historical* perspective. Hospices and palliative care have only a short history; but there is nevertheless a great deal to be learned from appraising that history when making sense of current and future dilemmas. In Part II of the book readers may wish to pay attention to the following four issues:

- The religious and philanthropical roots of the pre- and proto-hospices of the late nineteenth and early twentieth centuries.
- The rapid expansion of hospice and palliative care after 1967, giving rise to a need for more clarity of definition concerning the form and content of palliative care and the settings in which it is delivered.
- The emergence of a new subjectivity in late twentieth-century health care which extends clinical interest beyond the physical to encompass the psychological, social and spiritual dimensions of the patient's experience; this is linked in particular to new ideologies of the 'good death'.
- The suggestion that hospice and palliative care expansion has brought with it two penalties: routinization and medicalization.

Hospices have existed since early times, but it appears that it is only since the mid-nineteenth century that they have been concerned specifically with the care of the dying. The pre- and protohospices of the late Victorian and Edwardian eras had certain common features, being concerned mainly for the care of the dying poor in the urban areas. They combined a number of aspects: religious, philanthropic, moral and medical. Although several were established in the United Kingdom by the time of the First World War, they were not to develop in significant numbers for over half a century.

The welfare state of Britain in the post-Second World War era offered care 'from the cradle to the grave'. Preoccupied with acute and chronic health problems in a period of post-war social and economic reconstruction, it gave little emphasis however to the care of the dying. Nevertheless, changing demographic and epidemiological trends, concerns about the family and the care of the elderly, and new forms of medical specialization (e.g. in pain, geriatrics, psychiatry) all provided a stimulus to innovative thinking about the care of the dying. This was an era in which death was moving from the home to the hospital and where new evidence was coming to light of the poor home circumstances of elderly people, especially those with cancer. New charitable initiatives began to develop, such as the Marie Curie nursing homes, and several reports drew public attention to the needs of the dying.

It was of course the individual achievements of Cicely Saunders within this wider context which did so much to promote new ideas about the care of the dying. She was to replace the resignation of 'there is nothing more that we can do' with a new, positive approach to terminal care. She showed how with such an approach it was possible not only to overcome physical problems of pain and symptom management, but also to address the more intangible sufferings associated with social isolation, spiritual concerns and mental distress. From qualifying as a doctor in 1957 (after previous careers as a nurse and almoner) to the opening of St Christopher's in 1967, Cicely Saunders set out a remarkably detailed agenda for hospice care, including the specifics of its practice, but also the manner of its organization. Three factors seemed to have made this possible: a strong sense of personal calling to the work; a determined effort to raise the profile of terminal care on the professional agendas of doctors, nurses, social workers and others; and the active use of powerful social networks within the British establishment to give support to the enterprise.

By such means the basis was laid for a hospice movement which would quickly spread throughout the United Kingdom, and which would soon take on global proportions. With geographic spread also came diversification: from in-patient units, to home care, to day care and hospital-based services.

The expansion and broadening of services created a growing interest in the definition of 'hospice', 'terminal' and 'palliative' care and we also deal in Part II with some of these questions. The notion of 'palliation' has both positive and negative associations and the etymology of the term continues to be relevant to present-day definitions. Some early hospice writers made the distinction between 'cure' and 'care' but more recent 'models' of palliative care have emphasized that the palliative approach also has its place alongside active, curative treatment and at earlier stages of the disease process. It is this broadening of the scope of palliative care which is feared by some as a sign of losing the specific focus and special qualities of terminal care at the very end of life. Much professional commentary has gone into these issues and we explore this in detail. Readers should note that 'terminal care' was the common usage at least up to the late 1960s, when hospice care became a frequently used term; the use of 'palliative care' does not occur with any frequency until the late 1980s. In general our usage here reflects the time period to which we are referring.

Closely linked to the developing practice of hospice and palliative care have been ideas associated with 'the good death'. Some historians have argued that it was a particular feature of modern death in the twentieth century that it became impersonal, technological and dominated by professionals. Death in the hospital became the exemplar of this. New ideologies of the good death should be seen as a reaction to it. As we saw in Part I, such ideologies are closely bound up with the prevailing conditions of late modern culture. They involve notions of 'open awareness', 'truth telling', the expression of feelings and a sense of meaning and trust. Such ideologies must also be seen as evidence of a new subjectivity within health care practice, where patients are assessed not just for their physical symptoms and needs, but also in relation to their personal, psychological and spiritual concerns.

By such means it is possible to see how the concerns of palliative care connect with a broader set of issues within health care, going well beyond the portals of hospices and specialist palliative care units. Inevitably this has meant that the reformist ideologies of palliative care have been subjected increasingly to more critical scrutiny. Questions are now being asked about how well equipped the new specialty is to deal with the needs of large numbers of mainly older people, dying from non-malignant conditions. There are also issues, given the continuing predominance of hospital deaths, about how palliative care can take root effectively in that setting. Palliative care has expanded the volume of its activity and the scope of its patient group, but the implications of such a rapid expansion are still being assessed.

Certainly, some dissenting voices have been heard and we identify two areas where criticism has been most notable. The first contains the argument that the original aims and goals of the hospice movement are being 'routinized' and 'bureaucratized'. This position draws on the thinking of Max Weber about how social movements are inevitably transmuted, if they are to survive, into the iron cage of bureaucracy, where they become rule-bound and mechanistic in character. There is of course evidence that this is happening to hospices to some extent, but we are not convinced that the argument is based on solid historical evidence or that it signals an inevitable process. Second, and linked to the routinization thesis, are allegations about the creeping medicalization of palliative care. Again there is considerable evidence that medicine has become more involved in shaping the development of palliative care, but we are not convinced by romantically inclined commentators who suggest that this is something set to undermine the 'original' philosophy. Such commentary in our view frequently relies on a partial and simplistic account of what the 'original' stimuli to hospice developments actually were. In the British context at least, as evidenced by the early writings of Cicely Saunders (Clark 1998b), these were certainly heavily caught up with the need to *improve and extend* medical care at the end of life. The debate of course was around the precise form which this medicine should take.

Part II of the book therefore seeks to provide an overview of the historical development of hospice and palliative care. We show how within a period of only 30 years rapid expansion took place in the delivery of services and how the emerging specialty faced the issue of managing its boundaries in relation to the wider health care system. Expansion has brought growing concerns about the precise character of palliative care, about where it begins and ends and its place within late modern systems of health and social care delivery. Debates about routinization and medicalization also show how hospice ideals have wider resonances within late modern culture such that when these ideals are perceived to be threatened or compromised in some way, they give rise to a wider sense of public anxiety and concern. Part II should therefore be read for its focus upon the nineteenth-century origins of hospices in philanthropy, religion and medicine; for an attempt to characterize the broad parameters of palliative care philosophy and practice; for a discussion of the new subjectivity to be found in late twentieth-century health care, particularly as it relates to ideas about the 'good death'; and for a discussion of the putative 'routinization' and 'medicalization' of hospice and palliative care.

4 History and development

There is a liking among some of those who write about the historical development of palliative care to trace back the institutional origins of hospices to very early times. Thus Seplowin and Seravalli (1983) make links with special places which were used to contain plague victims in twelfth-century BC Greece. Likewise, various commentators (Corr and Corr 1983; Kastenbaum 1991) refer to Fabiola's shelters for travellers and sick people, whom she nursed in Rome in the fifth century AD. It was this notion of hospice that gained currency in mediaeval Europe, deriving from the Latin word *hospes*, which came to denote hospitality, particularly to strangers. Such institutions proliferated and according to McNulty and Holderby (1983) there were 750 of them in England by the thirteenth century.

Whilst the shared name speaks to a connection between these early institutions and the hospices of the modern era, we should be cautious in making too many direct comparisons between the two. For as the medical historian Roy Porter points out:

> In mediaeval England and throughout rural parts of continental Europe, hospices routinely provided care and hospitality for the indigent, elderly, infirm and for pilgrims, without predominantly being devoted to the sick.
>
> (Porter 1996: 210)

Similarly, Saunders notes:

> ... the mediaeval hospice was not primarily associated with dying people, and over the centuries it had come to welcome an impossible mix of patients alongside travellers and pilgrims, orphans, and the destitute with varying degrees of segregation.
>
> (Saunders 1993: vi)

The early hospices then were the generic forerunners to later systems of care for the dependent, the sick, the poor and the dying. In retaining the name, modern hospices have sought self-consciously to rekindle the tradition of devotion, calling and the ethic of service which was enshrined in the religious foundations of their predecessors. The idea that hospices, as places concerned specifically with the care of the dying, have a history stretching back into early times is however misleading and serves little purpose in advancing our understanding of such care in the past. It does, however, reveal something of the preoccupations of the modern hospice movement, which has developed a discourse of its history as something concerned with journeying, pilgrimage and the meaning of suffering.

The reformations of Henry VIII and Edward VI (1536–52) saw the dissolution of most religious hospitals and related foundations. In London small numbers were reinstated on a secular basis: St Bartholomew's and St Thomas's for the sick poor and Bethlem for the insane. Beyond this the country was hardly served at all and there were no other medical hospitals in England in 1700 (Porter 1996: 212). The age of enlightenment however saw the beginnings of hospital growth and new places sprang up to serve the respectable and deserving poor; paupers though were catered for under the terms of the Poor Law and suffered the indignities of the workhouse. Five new general hospitals appeared in London between 1720 and 1750 and others were opened in the provinces.

It is with the century that follows that Michel Foucault opens his analytical opus on *The Birth of the Clinic* (1973). For in the next hundred years medicine moved from the 'old myths of nervous pathology' to 'an era from which we have not yet emerged' (1973: x). Here was the beginning of the new *positive science* of medicine which took as its elements the physical examination, pathological anatomy and the codification of information in statistical form. This, as Foucault so graphically describes it, marked the shift to a new, all-encompassing clinical gaze:

> This new structure is indicated – but not, of course, exhausted – by the minute but decisive change, whereby the question: 'What is the matter with you?' with which the eighteenth century dialogue between doctor and patient began (a dialogue possessing its own grammar and style), was replaced by that other question: 'Where does it hurt?', in which we recognise the operation of the clinic and the principle of its entire discourse.
>
> (Foucault 1973: xviii)

Numbers of important developments were conjoined with the rise of modern medicine. Hospitals proliferated, often with medical men taking the initiative in their establishment, which served in turn as a stimulus to professional advancement. Specialist hospitals began to take off, including some which would later have important links with the rise of modern palliative care, such as, in London, the Brompton Hospital (1841) and the Royal Marsden Hospital (1851). This was also the era when the teaching hospitals were established and in which the Nightingale nursing reforms took place, with the first nurses to be trained under the new system commencing at St Thomas's in 1860.

It is in the nineteenth century also that we observe a rapid expansion in the medical division of labour. Within this occurred a growing differentiation about those places where the sick and dying were treated and cared for. In the new hospitals there was a growing emphasis upon curing those with acute illness. The chronic sick, the aged and the dying, and above all the poor, were scarcely welcome in the voluntary hospitals. As Porter observes: '. . . there was a medical screening process, which barred patients suffering from chronic, terminal or infectious conditions, for which the hospital could do nothing' (1989: 165). Such a procedure was designed to 'maximise bed-room for conditions which could profitably be treated – scurvy, abscesses, burns, skin complaints, leg ulcers, rheumatism, broken limbs, and the like' (Porter 1989: 165). As they emerged, therefore, the new hospices of the modern era combined an explicit focus on the care of the dying with particular attention to the poor.

Late nineteenth- and early twentieth-century hospices

There exists only a brief secondary literature on the early history of the modern hospices. Goldin (1981), though not specific, indicates that the first nineteenth-century hospice for the dying was opened in the 1830s in Australia, where it was attached to St Vincent's Hospital. Saunders, however, suggests that the first use of the word 'hospice', solely as a place for the dying, occurred a few years later in France, when Mme Jeanne Garnier opened the first of several *hospices* or *calvaires* (Saunders 1993). Both of these claims merit further investigation.

Most attention has focused on Our Lady's Hospice for the Dying which opened at Harold's Cross, Dublin in 1879. For Kerr (1993: 13) this was a 'defining moment in hospice history'. The hospice opened 21 years after the death of Mother Mary Aikenhead, founder of the Irish congregation of the Sisters of Charity, in the convent where she had died. From modest beginnings, the work extended in 1888 into purpose-built accommodation for 110 patients. Expansion to other places soon followed. The congregation established the Sacred Heart Hospice in Sydney, Australia in 1890. Fifteen years after that, in 1905, St Joseph's Hospice was opened in Hackney, in the east end of London.

Parallel developments were also taking place. The Free Home for the Dying, also known as the Hostel of God, was established in 1891, in Clapham, London, through a joint appeal between William Hoare, a philanthropic brewer, and the Anglican Order, St James's Servants of the Poor. Three years later Howard Barrett founded St Luke's House, near Regent's Park in London, where he served as part-time medical officer. St Luke's, in the view of Goldin, writing in 1981, '. . . was more than a prehospice. To a far greater degree than any institution of its time in London, caring primarily for the dying, it was a protohospice, using the word *hospice* in its contemporary sense' (Goldin 1981: 385).

Of particular interest in this period is the work of St Columba's Hospital or Home of Peace. This opened in 1889 and was based on the idea of a *Friedenheim*, developed in Germany as a place for the peaceful care of terminally ill tuberculosis patients. Now the concept was adapted to those with terminal cancer. Briefly it appeared that it might proliferate, but as Murphy points out:

> The cancer hospitals in three of Britain's largest industrial cities planned to open such homes in the country, where their patients would go, not to convalesce, but to die in peace and comfort. While all three hospitals did increase their provision for surgical treatment, none of them ever opened a Friedenheim. As belief in the new, more aggressive surgery strengthened, and the methods of physiological research repeatedly proved their success in the control of infectious diseases, investment in homes for the hopeless seemed increasingly inappropriate.
>
> (Murphy 1989: 227)

The building which had contained Britain's first, and only, Friedenheim was closed in 1985, demolished to make way for a Civic Centre at Swiss Cottage, London.

These hospices of the late nineteenth century, together with a small number of others which endured for shorter periods, pre-figure the wider developments which took place in the second half of the twentieth century. The pre- or protohospices have several features in common. They combined concerns which were religious, philanthropic, moral and medical.

Female religious orders expanded rapidly in the nineteenth century; care of the dying, in the case of the Sisters of Charity, was just one aspect of a wider set of concerns held by these orders which encompassed relief of the poor, service in the community and education. As Kerr puts it: 'Our Lady's Hospice for the Dying was a residential facility providing nursing and spiritual care, with limited medical service' (1993: 19). The care it offered was born of a religious tradition which accepted a measure of suffering in this world, just as it anticipated release in the next.

Philanthropy was important to all of the hospices, each of which came to rely on public and private subscriptions. Philanthropic service by women in England and Ireland in the nineteenth century has been described by Prochaska (1980) and Luddy (1995) respectively. Both reveal the importance of voluntary effort as a Christian duty, but also as a form of social control designed to impose middle-class behaviours and norms on the poor. Work in progress by Humphreys will cast light on the extent to which this extended even to the regulation of dying itself (Humphreys, in progress). Goldin makes clear that admission to St Luke's was unlikely for those who had received relief from the parish; this was a place for the 'deserving' poor (Goldin 1981). In this St Luke's appears to differ from the hospices run by the Sisters of Charity, for whom service to the poorest elements of society was (and remains) a central mission.

The wider medical debates surrounding the nineteenth-century homes for the dying lie beyond the scope of this chapter. Medical involvement (with the exception of St Luke's) was however limited and it was not until the middle of the next century that this was further developed. Of particular importance however was the fact that the homes were to be unequivocally for those close to death. Such a prerequisite might therefore make them unattractive to doctors involved in the curatively-oriented new hospital medicine system.

These homes for the dying established in the later years of the Victorian era therefore appear precariously poised. Rooted in religious and philanthropic concerns which would diminish after the First World War, their potential to develop appeared limited. In the event it was the changing medical construction of the dying process which would rekindle interest in the hospice as a separate institution of care and it was not until the 1950s that this process began to take shape. Most of the nineteenth- and early twentieth-century hospices were still in existence after the Second World War; for some of these a revolution in the theory and practice of caring for the dying was about to take place.

A movement originates

One of the paradoxes of the history of the modern hospice movement in Britain is that it was to originate in the shadow of a new, inclusive system of socialized medicine and welfare which would care for all in need, 'from the cradle to the grave'; we return to this in Chapter 7. Like the voluntary hospices which had preceded it, however, the priorities of the British National Health Service, established in 1948, were with acute illness and rehabilitation. This, coupled with an ideological rejection of charity as the appropriate source for the provision of health care, did not create an auspicious environment in which voluntary hospices might be expected to develop. Murphy notes that when Aneurin Bevan presented the NHS Bill to the British parliament he described how he would 'rather be kept alive in the efficient if cold altruism of a large hospital than expire in a gush of warm sympathy in a small one' (quoted in Murphy 1989: 234).

Webster sets out the challenges which faced the new National Health Service in Britain:

> In the first decade of the NHS it was necessary to convert a defective and ramshackle collection of inherited medical services into a modern health service appropriate to the needs and expectations of the second part of the twentieth century. The planners attempted this awesome task without anything like the material and human resources needed for the purpose. The scale of this operation was becoming ever greater owing to scientific advance, the rising capacities of medicine, changing demographic and epidemiological circumstances, and not least on account of rising aspirations; it was no longer reasonable to expect the less affluent classes to bear indignities associated with charity, the means test, poor relief, or inappropriate incarceration.
>
> (Webster 1996: 1)

Notwithstanding these difficulties, as Webster also notes, by the tenth anniversary of the NHS it was widely perceived to be a success story. In an era of post-war political consensus, both Conservative and Labour parties were open in their support for the new health service (Pierson 1996).

The detailed implications of this situation for developing concerns about the care of the dying are explored by one of us in a separate paper (Clark, in preparation). From this it can be seen that several factors were at work in influencing discourses on death and dying during the 1950s and it is these which provide the essential context for the development of the modern hospices. These factors include changing demographic and epidemiological trends; concerns about the family and the care of elderly people; and medical specialization.

During the 1950s the population was expanding. The birth rate had risen after the war (albeit only temporarily) but elderly people were also increasing as a portion of the population. By 1951 more than 10 per cent of the population was over 65 years, compared to less than 5 per cent in 1901 (Clarke 1996). It was also the era which marked a shift away from high mortality associated with infectious disease and the beginnings of a profile of chronic illness and disability among an ageing population. In this context there was growing interest in the problems associated with cancer. In 1951 the Marie Curie Memorial Foundation (a newly established cancer charity) and the Queen's Institute of District Nursing conducted a survey of 7000 cancer patients living at home. Their report (Marie Curie Memorial Foundation 1952) highlighted widespread problems, impoverished material circumstances and the need for improved institutional care. By the end of the decade there were few visible signs of improvement. The Marie Curie Memorial Foundation had gone on to open a number of nursing homes around the country, but a survey of homes for the dying, conducted by Dr H.L. Glyn Hughes, was somewhat critical of prevailing conditions.

His report, *Peace at the Last* (Glyn Hughes 1960), spoke of good intentions, but weakly developed technique in the terminal care homes of the day. Interestingly, the work being undertaken at St Joseph's, Hackney (although not named as such in the report) was singled out for particular praise.

Peace at the Last emphasized the desirability of care in the home wherever possible, but by the 1950s there were debates about the extent to which families were willing to support their sick, dependent and dying. Under the post-war programme of housing construction, large sections of the population were moved to new towns and suburban estates and there were concerns about the breakdown of traditional communities and family networks of support (Finch and Summerfield 1991). By 1956 40 per cent of deaths were occurring in NHS hospitals. Glyn Hughes recommended the combined virtues of 'a homely atmosphere' together with 'modern hospital surroundings and procedures' as the best way forward (1960: 31).

By the time of the publication of Glyn Hughes's report there was some evidence of an awakening medical interest in matters relating to the care of dying people. For example Exton-Smith had been undertaking work on the terminal illnesses of 220 geriatric patients, recording pain levels and awareness of dying (Exton-Smith 1961). Around the same time (1959–61), the psychiatrist John Hinton was conducting investigations aimed at assessing levels of physical and mental distress associated with terminal illness and seeking links between these and patients' personal lives (Hinton 1963). Another study (Aitken-Swann 1959) had focused on nursing patients with advanced cancer at home. Coupled to these we see the beginnings of medical specialization in geriatrics and in the study of pain, both of which start to expand in the course of the 1950s. Taken together such developments provide a context for understanding the specific contribution of one individual, Cicely Saunders.

The work of Cicely Saunders in the 1950s and 1960s is now being described in detail (Clark 1997a, 1998a, 1998b). Some aspects of her biography are well known (du Boulay 1984). Undergraduate years at Oxford were interrupted by war and followed by three years of nurse training at St Thomas's Hospital, London. Chronic back problems forced her to foreclose on a nursing career, however, after which she trained as a hospital almoner (or medical social worker in today's language). Caring for a dying Jewish émigré from Poland awakened her concerns about the special needs of dying patients. The patient in question, David Tasma, died in February 1948, just months before the foundation of the National Health Service, and leaving Cicely Saunders with a personal sense of wider work to be done. She began working as a volunteer at St Luke's, now in Bayswater, and still one of only a handful of homes for the dying in London. By the early 1950s she had been persuaded to undertake a third career path, in medicine. Returning to St Thomas's, she qualified as a doctor in 1957.

Whilst still a medical student she produced her first paper, published in the St Thomas's Hospital *Gazette* (Saunders 1958). Focusing on four patients with terminal cancer, the paper remains a remarkably far-sighted exposition of ideas which subsequently became so central to modern palliative care. Placed in the context of a discussion of the value of special homes for dying people, the paper considers in turn questions of nursing care, the terminal stage of disease, and pain, emphasizing the need for good physical care to be combined with psychological and spiritual assistance. There followed many more publications (Clark 1997a, 1998a), over 50 during the next decade alone (Clark 1998b). In these we can see Cicely Saunders working out the principles of a new approach to the care of dying people which would harness together medical innovation in pain and symptom management with wider concerns for the practical and social needs of patients and families, as well as a responsiveness to spiritual matters.

This clinical and intellectual agenda was pursued in parallel with a campaign to open the world's first modern hospice (Clark 1998a). In the second half of 1959 Cicely Saunders wrote to a handful of key individuals, setting out her ideas for what soon came to be called St Christopher's Hospice – the name was chosen deliberately to reflect the notion of journeying. By now she was deepening her knowledge of hospice organization through an extended period as a medical researcher at St Joseph's in Hackney. The new hospice plans took shape in detail: numbers of beds, architect's drawings, funding arrangements. From the outset St Christopher's was conceived as something separate from the NHS, but closely allied to it. A sustained fund-raising campaign was necessary, which eventually became national and international in character, drawing financial support from many countries. The opening of St Christopher's Hospice, in Sydenham, South London on 24 July 1967 was a huge practical accomplishment on the part of a woman who had passed through two careers before finally coming to medicine in mid-life.

Three sets of factors are crucial in explaining the achievement of Cicely Saunders during these early years (Clark 1998a). First, there is a powerful sense of personal calling which underpins her work. This emerges first as an individual vocation to work with dying people, but gradually is transmuted into a more generalized sense of the St Christopher's project being something divinely guided and inspired. Matters of the spirit, and of Christianity in particular, thus have a crucial influence on the development of hospice thinking from the outset. Second, there is the pursuit of a set of goals concerning the professional issues which relate to care of the dying. Publication plays a major part in this and a close reading of Cicely Saunders's writings at this time provides the sense of an unfolding professional and intellectual agenda. In the decade between writing her first paper and the opening of St Christopher's it is possible to detect both a deepening and a widening of the influences at work. Her papers gradually contain more references to other published work (as the related literature on death and dying expands). At the same time there is evidence of influences from many disciplines: medicine (particularly the new specialisms of pain, oncology and geriatrics), nursing, philosophy, theology, as well as the arts, humanities and social sciences. Whilst her ideas were *grounded* in modern medicine therefore, they were *elaborated* through a much wider, multidisciplinary discourse. In addition to the published articles and pamphlets written between 1957 and 1967, there was also a massive number of talks, lectures and public speaking engagements, through which her ideas were disseminated, in Britain, the United States and several European countries. Third, there were the social networks which had to be exploited to gain support for St Christopher's, particularly within the British establishment. Here we see the endorsement of senior figures in the world of politics, the law and the church; medical endorsement at the highest level proved peculiarly difficult to capture however.

It has been concluded from this (Clark 1998a) that from as early as the late 1950s Cicely Saunders had some sense that her ideas would not be restricted to the development of a single home for the dying, but might be disseminated and developed much further afield. As the project surrounding St Christopher's matured, Cicely Saunders became associated with a 'nascent movement' (Clark 1998a: 58) which would quickly spread to many other settings, and not only within the United Kingdom.

Global spread and redefinition

The global spread of hospices after 1967 has yet to be subject to rigorous historical or sociological enquiry. Together with related developments in palliative care it does of course continue to occupy the attention of many commentators who are caught up in the present-day implications of this work. Hospices and palliative care in this sense are matters of near history. Studying these subjects is therefore a process of reflexive engagement between perceptions of the past and preoccupations of the present. It is also important to acknowledge that the period after 1967 has been one of extremely rapid expansion and diversification. At the time of the opening of St Christopher's neither the term 'hospice movement' nor the description 'palliative care' were in use.

The spread of hospice ideas and practice in the United Kingdom and Ireland can be demonstrated relatively easily. Figure 4.1, based on data collected over a number of years by the Hospice Information Service, shows the growth of services in the British and Irish contexts.

Two things stand out in this figure. First, as Jackson and Eve (1997: 144) put it: 'The first decade of the modern hospice movement saw a steady increase in the number of hospices, but this growth was almost exclusively

Figure 4.1   Growth of palliative care services in the UK

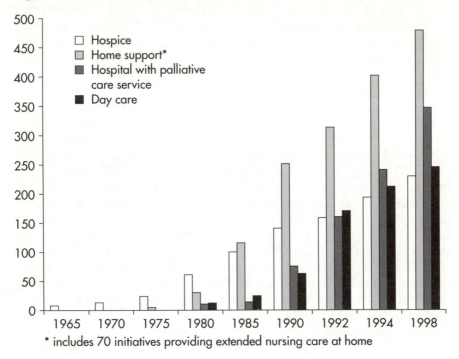

* includes 70 initiatives providing extended nursing care at home

Source: Hospice Information Service

confined to inpatient hospice services'. There were several reasons for this. Of primary importance was the fact that the developments were occurring in the charitable sector. The first modern hospices were driven exclusively by groups of local people who, under the framework of charitable organization, sought to promote the need for hospice care within their localities. Using St Christopher's as a model, the concept of a physical building was an important part of this vision. The bricks and mortar of a hospice building could be promoted to the local community and had an appeal to fund-raisers who might use the idea to stimulate charitable giving in various ways. So it was that by the early 1970s hospices were beginning to appear in different parts of the United Kingdom. The first of these were St Luke's, Sheffield, which was designed by the same architect as St Christopher's, and St Anne's, in Manchester, both of which opened in 1971.

In-patient care was also the focus of attention for another reason. At this stage hospices were concerned unequivocally with terminal care. Their purpose was often seen as that of providing a sensitive and gentle environment in which people could die peacefully. In that sense they were construed as an alternative to the busy, technical atmosphere of the modern hospital. Accordingly, the idea of physical separation from the mainstream of health care services was an important notion to the founders of modern hospices. By 1975, however, a change began to occur in this pattern of independent hospice development. In that year the first purpose-built 'continuing care' unit was opened in the grounds of a general hospital. This brought hospice practice into close proximity with hospital care, but again there was a strong input from charitable sources. The continuing care units were designed and built with support from the then National Society for Cancer Relief, but running costs became the responsibility of the NHS. In total about a dozen continuing care units were to be developed using this model.

The second important feature displayed in Figure 4.1 however is the pattern of diversification which is revealed. Certainly the initial attention was given to in-patient units, but developments quickly occurred in other settings. In 1969 St Christopher's Hospice began a home care service which would take hospice skills and philosophy into the wider community. The most important manifestation of this approach however came in the work of specially selected and trained Macmillan Nurses, who first began to appear in the mid-1970s. Again these were funded initially by the Macmillan charity, most usually on an initial pump-priming basis, after which the costs would be met by the health service. Macmillan Nurses began to provide specialist advice, guidance and education to members of the primary health care teams. In this way they added to the range of services available to terminally ill people in the community. In particular the Macmillan Nurses could complement the service provided by another charity, the Marie Curie Foundation, which since the late 1950s had been providing home nursing, especially at night, for patients at the end of life. Jackson and Eve (1997) indicate that by the mid-1990s there were over 1000 Macmillan Nurses, approximately 400 home care teams and some 5000 Marie Curie Nurses in the United Kingdom.

Similar developments have taken place in hospitals. A specialist support team working in hospital first appeared in Britain in 1976, at St Thomas's Hospital, and was similar to one started two years earlier in St Luke's Hospital, New York. These multi-professional teams comprise doctors, nurses, social worker, chaplain and secretary. They focus on pain and symptom management as well as emotional support to patients and caregivers. Other developments in hospital have included individual nurses, or small teams of nurses providing specialist care and expertise.

Finally, an additional element of the expansion of services is in the provision of day care. First started at St Luke's Hospice, Sheffield, in 1975, and conceived of as 'a day out for the patient and a day off for the carer' (Cockburn and Twine 1982: 1410), the day units burgeoned to over 200 programmes in the UK by the late 1990s. Attendance at day care could provide opportunities for pain and symptom management, but is often likely to emphasize the social and personal needs of the patient, focusing on therapeutic activities of various kinds, including painting, crafts, poetry, reminiscence, whilst also providing opportunities for massage, hair care and so on.

In the United Kingdom therefore expansion in services has proceeded rapidly over a 30-year period. The sustainability of that expansion is a question to which we will turn in a later chapter. Expansion has also been a feature of hospice and palliative care services in other parts of the world, though in each context the timing and rate of growth has varied. In particular the forms and settings in which this type of care is delivered vary greatly from country to country. Whilst the 'British model' is often referred to in discussions, it should not be assumed that this is an approach which can or should be adopted elsewhere. The global spread of hospice and palliative care is associated with a large measure of local variation, though some underlying common threads and challenges also appear (we will address these in the next chapter). In a book of this kind it is possible only to offer a brief sketch, from secondary sources, of key developments around the world; this is again a topic which merits more detailed study.

Rather than viewing the development of St Christopher's Hospice as a stone dropped into a pond, creating ripples which eventually spread around the globe, it is preferable to consider a different metaphor. Something horticultural might suffice. Global hospice and palliative care developments might be seen, for instance, as a series of orchards. These have been planted differently according to local aspect and conditions, and they may favour particular species which differ from place to place. Likewise, methods of cultivation may vary. Linking the orchards however may be certain rootstock or cultivars which are common to most places, and of course there is a great deal of cross-pollination, created by visitors who move from one orchard to another, dispersing pollen and creating hybrid vigour. In this way the hospice and palliative care orchard has extended, sometimes drawing on ancient rootstock, but also producing new varieties from time to time.

As Kastenbaum notes, in 1973 there were no hospice programmes in the United States; by the late 1990s there were over 2000 (Kastenbaum 1997). Such rapid development he attributes to two important changes. The first of these was a growth, from the 1970s, in a form of consumerism concerned with a rediscovery of 'the natural': in food, lifestyle, leisure, health care; even death care. The second influence was the rising interest in thanatological subjects among academics, professionals and the wider public. Together, he argues, these had an influence on the prevailing 'death system' in the United States, reversing a secular decline in attention to care of the dying person, the disposal of the dead and social consolidation following death. As Small (1997a) has noted, the rise of hospice in the United States can be construed as a reaction against the medicalization of death. Accordingly hospice programmes in that country have had a strong emphasis upon social models of care; they have been focused on care in the home rather than in institutions; and they rely heavily on the involvement of nurses and volunteers, rather than doctors.

Two related events changed the direction of American hospice in the 1980s. First, the claims of hospice protagonists were assessed through a demonstration project (Mor *et al.* 1988). Known as the National Hospice Study, USA, the project collected data from 40 hospice and 14 conventional care programmes. Among the 833 hospice home care patients, 624 hospice in-patients and 297 conventional care patients who participated, it was found that the hospice services used fewer expensive and invasive medical procedures and that the patients spent longer at home. Hospice in-patients tended to score more favourably on pain, symptoms and satisfaction with care among family members. Hospice home care was cheaper than conventional care, but for both hospice in-patients and hospice care patients, the longer they remained in the programme, the less a cost saving was demonstrated against conventional care.

The second key event was the recognition of hospice care by the United States Medicaid system, a process influenced in part by the National Hospice Study findings. From 1982 this provided a foundation of economic support for hospice programmes. As Kastenbaum puts it: 'After two decades, hospice care has itself become part of the health system establishment that it once challenged' (1997: 107). Beresford (1993) has distinguished several models of hospice organization within the USA: community-based; home health agency-based; hospital-based; volunteer-intensive; freestanding. A growing trend is towards 'proprietary' hospices, which operate as profit-generating businesses and are bought and sold as commercial concerns.

The contrasting examples of hospice development in the UK and the USA are refracted and reflected in other settings. In some parts of the Commonwealth, or former colonies of the British Empire, the UK hospice model has had considerable influence. Hospices akin to those in Britain can thus be found in Southern Africa, New Zealand and Australia. At the same time, such hospices have often had particular priorities, born of local circumstances. For example, Island Hospice in Zimbabwe in its early days developed a bereavement service for those traumatized by a bloody war of independence (Buckland 1997). Elsewhere hospice developments have taken place, for example in Eastern Europe, in the shadow and aftermath of communism (Jujawska Tenner 1997; Luczak 1997).

The World Health Organisation's Cancer and Palliative Care Programme has cautioned against the unplanned spread of hospices, in favour of a public health-oriented approach which has prioritized cancer pain as a target for service developments. As Stjernsward puts it: 'Relief of suffering from terminal cancer is an urgent need that could be the spearhead, the model, for what can be done through a public health approach' (1997: 13–14). This strategy is concerned with the *dissemination* of existing knowledge, the *implementation* of government strategies to relieve suffering and the *mobilization* of resources to make pain-relieving drugs available easily and equitably. It is an approach which finds echoes in some first world countries and regions wishing to develop a more strategic approach to the provision of palliative care services. Thus in Catalonia, the emphasis has been on high coverage, through the deployment of palliative care teams in local health clinics, general hospitals and oncology centres (Gomez-Batiste *et al.* 1997).

Two recent compilations give substantial insights into the detailed development of hospice and palliative care around the world (Clark *et al.* 1997a; Saunders and Kastenbaum 1997). One significant landmark within these developments has been the emergence and recognition of palliative care as a specialty in its own right. The recognition of palliative medicine took place in Britain 1987. 'Palliative care' is a term used increasingly in preference to 'hospice care' in many countries. Disentangling the nomenclature and its implications is a major current preoccupation of the specialty. Just as the history of the modern hospice and palliative care movement is beginning to be written, therefore, so too we are seeing a widening debate about the limits and boundaries to this burgeoning specialty. It is to these questions that we now turn.

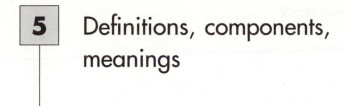

5 | Definitions, components, meanings

As palliative care has developed, so it has become associated with a widening range of terms. We have seen a shift from 'terminal care' to 'palliative care' (and/or 'palliative medicine'), as well as distinctions between 'specialist palliative care' and 'the palliative care approach'. The scope for confusion in the usage and application of these labels is clearly apparent and indicates the value of a close examination of their differences and similarities. The recent differentiation of terminology under the hospice and palliative care umbrella is, however, underpinned by shared cultural ideals about the ideal circumstances and 'way' of death. These cultural ideas may be described collectively as the ideology of the 'good death', and have been the subject of much recent debate and theorization among sociologists. Hospice and palliative care has, it might be argued, become synonymous with 'good death'. It stands now not only as a 'symbolic critique' (McNamara 1997: 3) of medicalized, institutionalized death, but has also become a central point of reference for popular expectations of dying and of standards of care at the time of death. These are, however, expectations which remain as yet unfulfilled for the vast majority of the dying population.

In this chapter we address each of these interrelated issues in turn. We provide an overview of the terms and concepts which constitute 'palliative care'; and then discuss the 'good death' ideal, showing how it is portrayed in a number of theoretical writings. We turn lastly to a critical analysis of the mismatch between the popular experience of death and dying, and the popular expectations surrounding those processes. Special attention is paid to the situation of older people who suffer from non-cancer disease and who thus fall outside the traditional remit of palliative care.

What is palliative care?

It is not uncommon among palliative care commentators to describe the origins of the word 'palliative' in the Latin verb *palliare*. This we are often told means 'to cloak or shield' and it is from this notion that modern palliative care takes its cue. This seems to us a deeply problematic etymological starting point for the new specialty and one which from the outset throws up contradictions and possibilities for varied interpretation. Some recent work, for example, has emphasized in a critical manner the concealment or disguising which is associated with the Latin noun *pallium*, meaning 'cloak' (Scott 1994; Lawton 1998). A helpful short article by Morris (1997) however gives the first serious attention we have seen to the sociolinguistic history of 'palliation' and in so doing sets out two contrasting interpretations.

Morris puts forward two 'rival histories' of palliation 'summarized through the figures of the cloak and the shield' (1997: 1). From the outset, he argues, palliation is associated in the medical lexicon, from its origins in Elizabethan England, with pejorative associations and quackery: cloaking, covering up and disguising symptoms, whilst leaving the disease untouched. From our own researches we can add some examples to this from the seventeenth- and eighteenth-century medical literature: 'They knew there followed nothing but palliations of diseases' (Biggs *New Dispensatory* 1651); 'He is but half a physician; he hath palliated our sores and diseases, but he hath not removed them (Sharp *Sermon* 1738).

It is these associations, Morris suggests, which derive from the Latin *palla*, a long outer garment worn by Roman women, and the Latin verb *pallio*, 'to conceal'. Thus Samuel Johnson in 1755 can define palliate as 'To cure imperfectly or temporarily, not radically; to ease, not cure' (Morris 1997: 1).

Set against this etymological root, with its negative and pejorative associations, lies an alternative which Morris identifies in the Indo-European linguistic tradition. Here 'palliate' derives from an earlier word, *pel*, which refers to an animal skin or hide. Now the Greeks constructed the *pelte* from such skins to create a shield – an animal skin stretched over a wooden frame. Here it seems lies the possibility of a more positive and creative metaphor. As Morris puts it:

> What benefits might flow from an etymology that replaces the cloak with the shield? The act of shielding or protecting the patient offers the care giver a more active and possibly even heroic role. It gives a benign twist to the military metaphors inescapable in Western biomedicine. It avoids the pejorative idea of merely covering over or covering up. It implies the need for skill and knowledge. It respects the reality of danger and the imperatives of watchfulness. The shield,

that is, signifies contingency as well as protection, weakness as well as
strength. We employ a shield because we anticipate injury. A shield,
moreover, does not address the prospect of a distant or theoretical harm.
It is designed to offer a measure of practical security amid circumstances full of risk and uncertainty. It affirms life at a time when life is
under threat.

(Morris 1997: 11)

Morris's reference to the notion of 'heroism' is interesting in relation to
our earlier discussion of late modern dying. No doubt arguments between
the cloak and the shield will continue to be played out in palliative care
commentary, though for the moment (and perhaps regrettably) it is the
former which holds sway.

The notion of palliative health care therefore tends to be associated with
the concealment and relief of distressing symptoms suffered by people who
have a disease that cannot be cured. As Doyle (1994) points out, such a
description might be applied to most of the work performed by all health
care professionals. Indeed the model on which contemporary medical practice is based encourages the paradigmatic view that disease consists of a
series of 'symptoms' exhibited by a patient. These must be addressed individually by means of a paternalistic and linear problem-solving approach
(Kearney 1992). How then may 'palliative care' be distinguished from
mainstream health care? We would argue that the alignment of 'palliative'
with 'care' is crucially important here. The concept of 'care' is the key
to understanding the philosophy which informs the practice, organization
and delivery of palliative interventions to seriously ill people and their companions. 'Care', which has become associated with a wealth of meanings
and resonances, may be described as the organizing concept in this field of
health provision. The concept of 'care' directs attention from paternalism to
participation, from linearity to holism, and, most importantly, from patient
to person. As Roy says, '. . . the governing idea of palliative and hospice
care has been: see, not just the patient, but the person in his totality and
total particularity' (Roy 1995: 19). 'Care' in this holistic context becomes
an activity encompassing the full range of tasks involved in caring for a
person. It is an indication of the nature of the relationship between people:
the respect and compassion involved in caring *about* a person. Palliative
caring thus offers a particular promise to seriously ill and dying people
and their companions. The promise is that of integration, in the face of
the profoundly disintegrative threat of life-threatening illness and death.
Buckingham (1996) puts it thus:

Historically . . . dying has been a coming-apart experience for most
families. [Palliative] care concentrates on making the process of dying
a coming together experience for patient and family . . .

(Buckingham 1996: bookcover)

Ahmedzai (1993) rightly makes the point that palliative care does not have a monopoly on 'caring' and that to suggest otherwise would be an affront to the efforts of those engaged within other models of health care delivery. 'Caring' and 'curing' are sometimes posited as mutually exclusive activities, but this is clearly false. Each is an integral part of the other. Caring is, of course, an important feature of 'curing' work. However, it might be argued that in the modernist arena of health care delivery, 'caring' is sometimes subsumed to the activities of treatment and disease management. This characteristic feature of contemporary health care becomes particularly problematic when the treatment of disease is complex, of an uncertain outcome, and endures over a long period of time. Such a description might be applied to much of the experience of serious ill health endured by older people and by people suffering from conditions such as HIV disease and AIDS. Here, death and dying are 'known' future prospects, but at an 'unknown' time. The journey towards death is punctuated by periods of acute, short-term, and reversible illness. These episodes become progressively closer and more difficult to treat. As Jennings and George state:

> . . . the extreme uncertainty of compound pathologies abolishes the distinctions between cure and palliation . . . [and] curable components within a progressive and fatal syndrome often leave one unclear when to begin drawing lines . . .
>
> (Jennings and George 1996: 44)

The division of labour between nursing and medicine demonstrates some of the tensions that are involved in achieving a balance between caring and curing activities. For example, Salvage makes the point that the recent successes of nurses in refashioning the organization of their work towards a more personalized, 'caring' model are undermined by 'the central predicament of nursing as a woman's occupation in a man's world [and] the traditional marginalisation of nursing by medicine and governments . . .' (1995: 274). One aspect of this 'traditional marginalisation' has been the very invisibility of work which focuses on the formation of essentially private, inter-subjective relationships. Numbers of empirical studies (Field 1989; Mackay 1993; Walby and Greenwell 1994) have demonstrated that the successful execution of nursing work is contingent upon contextual and structural circumstances that are largely beyond the influence of nurses but in which doctors exert considerable control. For example, in a comparative study of the nursing care delivered to dying patients in various settings Field (1989: 122) demonstrated clearly the difficulties facing nurses during the negotiation of the 'space' required for the implementation of those aspects of their work which are difficult for others to 'see' and for nurses themselves to articulate. Using terminology employed by Strauss *et al.* (1985), Field highlighted how the 'comfort' and 'sentimental' aspects of nursing work are embedded within the more visible activities of 'machine', 'safety' and 'articulation' work associated with the essentially medically controlled treatment of patients.

Palliative care is predicated upon a teamwork model in which these barriers between disciplines are said to be lowered, if not dismantled completely, although the extent to which this has been achieved has not, however, been subjected to critical scrutiny. What though are the essential principles contained within palliative care? Three elements stand out: 'total care'; 'teamwork' and trust.

'Total care' refers to the multidimensional relief of suffering (Cassell 1991) whether experienced by ill persons or by their companions; 'teamwork' alludes to the model of interdisciplinary working required for effective palliative care; and 'trust' is about the nature of the relationship between the cared-for person and his/her carers – a relationship in which mutual autonomy is facilitated (Randall and Downie 1996). The alignment of these principles gives rise to some of the definitions of 'palliative care' currently available (cf. SMAC/SNMAC 1992; Higginson 1993; NCHSPCS 1994, 1995c). All of these are based to some degree on the definition set out by the World Health Organisation in 1990:

> Palliative care is the active total care of patients whose disease is not responsive to curative treatment. Control of pain, of other symptoms, and of psychological, social and spiritual problems is paramount. The goal of palliative care is achievement of the best possible quality of life for patients and their families. Many aspects of palliative care are also applicable earlier in the course of the illness, in conjunction with anti-cancer treatment. Palliative care:
>
> * affirms life and regards dying as a natural process
> * neither hastens nor postpones death
> * provides relief from pain and other distressing symptoms
> * integrates the psychological and spiritual aspects of patient care
> * offers a support system to help the family cope during the patient's illness and in their own bereavement.
>
> (WHO 1990)

As recently as 1980 'palliative care' was known as 'terminal care' and was firmly linked both to cancer services and to the period immediately before death. The terms remain, in common and sometimes interchangeable usage. How may we distinguish between these two terms, and at what stage does palliative care give way to terminal care?

Biswas (1993), in an analysis of recent changes in the delivery and organization of services to dying people, argues that

> . . . palliative care shifts the focus of attention away from death [but] there is real danger that by talking about and focusing upon palliation,

people may stop talking about and confronting the fact that the individual is going to die.

(Biswas 1993: 135)

There seems to be a concern here that the special focus of terminal care will
be obscured by the inclusion of 'all comers', many of whom may be months
or even years away from death. The National Council of Hospice and Specialist Care Services in a statement of definitions attempts to resolve this
dilemma by defining terminal care as part of palliative care:

> . . . [terminal care is] an important part of palliative care, and usually
> refers to the management of patients during the last few days or weeks
> or months of life from a point at which it becomes clear that the
> patient is in a progressive state of decline.
>
> (NCHSPCS 1995c: 5)

In this same document, people who are 'terminally ill' are defined as those
with '. . . active and progressive diseases for which curative treatment is
not possible or not appropriate and from which death can reasonably be
predicted within twelve months' (NCHSPCS 1995c: 5).

This usage of the term implies that the moment of transition from
'palliative' to 'terminal' is relatively clear, and that the length of remaining
life can be predicted with some accuracy. These are both issues for debate.
Further, some commentators argue that applying the label of 'terminal care'
to such a broad, loosely specified time span conveys an attitude towards
dying people that implies negativism and passivity. For example, Doyle
et al. point out that '. . . "terminal" suggests that all is finished, that there is
neither the time nor the opportunity to do more, and that active treatment
is unjustified and might well be undignified' (Doyle et al. 1993: 3).

O'Brien (1996) contends that it is this image which perpetuates the
habitual pattern of late referrals to palliative care programmes and the
notion of 'there is nothing more to be done'.

One way of addressing these problems of conceptual clarity has been
provided by the World Health Organisation committee report on cancer
pain relief and palliative care (1990). The report argues that curative and
palliative care are not mutually exclusive, and that palliative care should
become a gradually increasing part of an individual cancer sufferer's management. No differentiation is made between palliative care and terminal
care. A pragmatic distinction is made in the report between 'developed'
and 'developing' countries in recognition of the relative deprivation of the
latter, and a recommendation of the report is that developing countries
spend a greater proportion of their resources on palliative care rather than
on curative treatment. Higginson (1993: 6) notes that a major difficulty in
achieving a balance between curative treatment and palliative care is the
predominance of large-scale, randomized controlled trial research in the

Figure 5.1   'Sheffield' theoretical model for palliative care

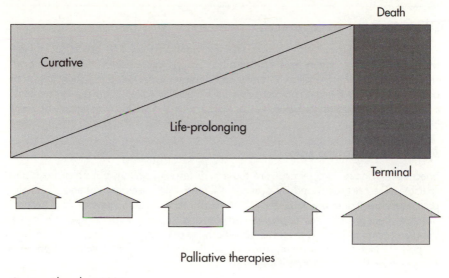

Source: Ahmedzai 1996

evaluation of cancer treatment. Here, there is a continuing, and almost exclusive, emphasis on length of life. The quality of life, death and the impact of cancer on the sufferer's companions are issues that are not addressed in such 'gold standard' investigations.

Ahmedzai (1996: 2) points out that most contemporary views, including the WHO model, of the interface between palliative care and curative care depend on the identification of the moment of 'critical transition' between the two. He argues that such a representation is both 'nihilistic and inaccurate' (1996: 2); first, because there is often no critical moment of transition and second, because 'curative' often means 'life prolonging' (as in the five- or ten-year survival rates used by oncologists as outcome measures), not recovery in the everyday sense of the word. Based on the identification of this distinction between 'curative' and 'life prolonging', Ahmedzai proposes a new conceptual model of palliative care, which emphasizes the intertwined nature of the various treatment and care modalities at *all stages* of the disease trajectory (see Figure 5.1).

This 'Sheffield' model makes a distinction between palliative care and terminal care based on a point at which adjuvant attempts either to prolong life or to give curative therapy are stopped, and therapies focused entirely on palliation remain. However, as Ahmedzai emphasizes, this should not entail negativism but rather a major shift in thinking about the purposes of care. Here, the prolongation of life (even if it is less than five years), the

Figure 5.2   Amalgamated definitions of palliative care

The palliative care approach

The palliative care approach aims to promote both physical and psychosocial well-being and is a vital and integral part of all clinical practice whatever the illness or its stage. It includes consideration of family and domestic carers. Management decisions can be guided by the patient's concerns and anxieties rather than purely medical/physical considerations. A palliative care approach should be a core skill of every clinician.

Specialist palliative care

Specialist palliative care services are those services with palliative care as their core specialty. They are delivered by professional staff with specialist training. Specialist palliative care teams are multidisciplinary and relate to both general and hospital practice, being available to provide advice and support that bridges the divide between home and hospital and to provide hospice care. Education, research, and support of other health care professionals giving care with a palliative care approach are key roles for specialist palliative care.

Palliative medicine

Palliative medicine refers to that contribution to the practice and study of palliative care which is made by doctors. It was recognized as a distinct field of medicine in 1987. Doyle *et al.* (1993) define palliative medicine as 'the study and management of patients with far advanced disease for whom the prognosis is limited and the focus of care is the quality of life'.

---

quality of remaining life and the quality of dying and death become ends in themselves; not indicators of failure or even second-best options.

The foregoing has attempted to clarify the meaning of palliative care and the distinctions between palliative care, terminal care, curative and life prolonging therapies. These are slippery concepts which, as we have shown, are subject to ongoing debate and reformulation. It is perhaps more straightforward to draw distinctions between the various terms which appear under the 'palliative care' umbrella. In Figure 5.2 we have amalgamated definitions put forward by Finlay and Jones (1995); the National Council for Hospice and Specialist Palliative Care Services (NCHSPCS 1995c, 1997c); and Gilbert (1996).

From these definitions we can see that a distinction may be made between the *delivery* of palliative care by professionals with specialist training in palliative care and the *philosophy* of palliative care as an element in the care delivered by non-specialist practitioners. A consultative document published by the National Council for Hospice and Specialist Palliative Care

Services (NCHSPCS 1994) makes a useful categorization of palliative care services which helps to clarify the distinction. Here it is suggested that palliative care services are a continuum of provision existing on three levels. The first level is characterized by the use of palliative care principles or 'approach', and may be discerned within general practitioner services or within long-term care institutions such as residential and nursing homes. The second level is characterized by the presence of trained and accredited specialist practitioners who use their skills during the course of their work in a range of non-specialist settings. The third level of provision is characterized by a high concentration of trained staff with access to a range of specialized expertise and in which services are provided either at home or in a specialist setting such as a hospice. Specialist palliative care services at the second and third levels are usually provided in addition to mainstream services, and where it has been decided that an individual patient will benefit from such specialist help. However, as Robbins points out, the label 'specialist palliative care' may be of dubious justification:

> If specialists actually provide something which non-specialists cannot or do not, then the label is probably justified. However, in the case of palliative care, it is not always clear what, in addition, specialists provide over non-specialists. Is it up-to-date knowledge of pharmacological and non-pharmacological advances in pain and symptom control? Is it counselling skills in breaking bad news, and effective communication? Is it practical advice on benefits and financial matters? Equally possible, could it be a matter of resources, such as *time* for unhurried consultations and nursing sessions, or *easily* accessible beds for respite and terminal care, or *effective* multidisciplinary team working?
>
> (Robbins 1997: 18)

It can be seen from the following discussion that the practice of palliative care is surrounded by some important etymological and definitional problems. Perhaps it is a key phase in the natural history of this emerging specialty that it should just now be so preoccupied with such matters. Undoubtedly discussion of these questions will help to clarify the aims and purposes of palliative care – and this will be essential to its continued expansion in an era which places increasing emphasis upon the evidence base of health care (Robbins 1998). At the same time, there is a danger that such debates can be inward-looking, self-referential and without impact on the mainstream of medicine and clinical practice. Despite these problems, there is undoubtedly one area of its work for which palliative care is now well known and where its contribution can readily be identified by insiders and outsiders alike. We refer here to the hospice and palliative care contribution to ideas about the 'good death', and it is to this issue that we now move on.

The 'good death'

As we have seen, the growth and development of contemporary palliative care is tied closely to the emergence of the modern hospice movement in the middle part of the twentieth century. Roy captures the strength of this association: 'Palliative and hospice care [were] conceived in the crucible of dying cancer patient neglect . . .' (1995: 19). Doyle in turn emphasizes the pivotal influence of the 'visionary genius' of Cicely Saunders who '. . . recognised need and acted to meet it, when others of us were either blind to it or saw it, but failed to act' (Doyle 1992). As we have seen, Saunders and her colleagues mounted an effective challenge to the assumptions guiding 'good' medical practice, by presenting both a conceptual critique *and* a workable, alternative model of delivering medical and nursing care to seriously ill and dying people. However, the roots of palliative care as a philosophy extend far beyond the pragmatic and compassionate concerns which were the driving force behind the emergence of the modern hospice movement. The notion of the 'good death' can be used to explore the variety of historical and philosophical influences which have converged into the recognizable patterning of ideas that constitute modern 'palliative care': ideas that have taken root in a variety of health care, academic and informal settings. Kellehear (1990) gives a succinct overview of the origins of the 'good death' concept, making a useful distinction between 'good death' in the sense of dying painlessly by means of euthanasia and 'good death' in the sense of adhering to a set of socially sanctioned modes of behaviour:

> Good death is a phrase created from the Greek 'Kalos Thanatos' rather than from another Greek source, 'Eu Thanatos'. The conceptual distinction derived from its etymological sources is important sociologically. As discussed here, Good Death is derived from Kalos Thanatos translating as 'beautiful death, the ideal or exemplary' death . . . 'Eu Thanatos' on the other hand, is often broadly but accurately translated as Good Death also. However, 'Good' in the 'Eu' sense, additionally refers to dying well, that is painlessly, easily . . . as in the broad meaning of euthanasia . . . Good Death in the Kalos sense is a set of culturally sanctioned and prescribed behaviours set in motion by the dying and designed to make death meaningful for as many concerned as possible . . .
>
> (Kellehear 1992: 29)

As Kellehear notes, prescribed behaviours and expected modes of 'being' surrounding death have been, and continue to be, an important and rich feature of cultural life within many different societies. Rees (1997), writing from the perspective of psychology, gives a comprehensive overview of the major world religions together with their associated mourning and funeral customs. He conjoins this overview with an analysis of the patterning of ideas about the significance of death within the huge variety of cultural and religious contexts that exist within contemporary life. In a more sociological vein, Field *et al.* (1997) explore differences in the way that death is experienced and expressed in various cultures and by men and women within those cultures. A central theme in their analysis is the crucial role of social context and wider cultural environment in shaping the meaning of what may be perceived as a private, individual encounter with death and dying.

In our Western culture, much of the literature and research concerning the modern 'way' and attitude to the constitution of good death contains a common, pervasive theme. In essence, this theme is that of a critique of hospitalized, medicalized death and its representation as a threat to an idealized good death. Hospitalized death, in this literature, is characterized by a loss of individual choice; fear; isolation from family, friends and professional carers; lack of knowledge about the dying state; and by a prolongation of the dying career. Lofland (1978) identified six defining features of contemporary death which combine powerfully to produce these experiences:

1 a high level of medical technology;
2 early disease detection;
3 a complex definition of death;
4 a high prevalence of chronic disease;
5 a low incidence of fatal injuries and
6 active intervention in the dying process.

It is possible to discern a romantic image in commentaries on death and dying, in which contemporary institutionalized death is portrayed as divorced increasingly from the 'traditional' good death of earlier times. Here death was a frequent visitor across the age range, and involved the immediate family and the wider community. Rituals associated with dying and with death were religious, prescriptive, and publicly acknowledged. They emphasized stability, the unchanging nature of the world and the certainty of an afterlife. Individual frailty did not matter ultimately because each person could relate to a greater, divine whole. Control over nature was seemingly impossible. Ariès put forward a thesis of 'tamed death' (1976: 1) to explain attitudes to death in the time period between the fifth and nineteenth centuries. Here, the fear of death was submerged within a sense of collective destiny and contained by the ritual behaviours with which it was surrounded. Ariès argued that such resignation and acceptance which characterized good death in pre-twentieth-century life have been replaced in the twentieth century by an overwhelming fear, a fear that has its roots in the individualistic principles on which modern life is based:

> The old attitude in which death was both familiar and near, evoking no
> great fear or awe, offers too marked a contrast to ours, where death is
> so frightful that we dare not utter its name.
>
> (Ariès 1976: 13)

Death thus came to be seen as something 'ugly' and intrinsically bad,
something which must be hidden from view to reduce its threat to social
order. Ariès traced the roots of the emergent sense of 'self-identity', in
which the identity of the group or community became secondary to that
of the individual, to cultural and religious changes which began in the
eleventh and twelfth centuries. He went on to describe how the social
and industrial revolutions of the nineteenth century confirmed death as
a metaphor for isolation and separation: 'Death became the unaccepted
separation, the death of the other, "thy death", the death of the loved one'
(Ariès 1976: 106).

This separation was strengthened by an emergence of medical–technical
involvement in everyday lives that ensured the physical removal of dying
people from their homes to a bureaucratic, specialized and segmented
institution: the hospital. Here death was '. . . dissected, cut to bits by a
series of little steps, which makes it impossible to know which step was the
real death' (1976: 88), and by the involvement of impersonal experts who
stood in judgement over the status and condition of one particular part of
the body.

In Ariès's thesis, death has disappeared from community life and communal awareness and been relocated as an individual experience occurring within the defining power of the medical expert. Further, it has been
accompanied by a profound alteration in societal attitudes. In these, death
loses its 'everyday' quality and becomes that which is mysterious, meaningless and feared. Other commentators support Ariès's claim; thus Gorer
(1965) refers to the contemporary 'taboo' or 'pornography' of death, while
Mellor and Shilling (1994) refer to a contemporary 'sequestration' of death
characterized by a lack of ability to ascribe meaning to it. As we saw in
Chapter 1, they draw on Giddens's concept of 'ontological security' (1991)
and Elias's concept of 'lonely' dying (1985), to describe how

> . . . modernity has not just emptied the sky of angels but has emptied
> tradition, ritual and increasingly, virtually all overarching normative
> meaning structures of their content . . . the reduction of the scope of the
> sacred from the wider cosmos to the area of the individual existence
> mirrors the transference of the significance of death from the social
> body to the individual body, a general privatisation of meaning and
> experience, leaving individuals alone to construct and maintain values
> to guide them through life and death, a situation prone to reality
> threatening ontological and existential anxieties.
>
> (Mellor and Shilling 1994: 428–9)

Bauman (1992) suggests that contemporary society has organized itself on the basis of trying to avoid death. He identifies two strategies which are employed to ward off 'the problem' of death. The first strategy attempts to 'deconstruct' death into individual problems of health and disease which are potentially soluble given enough adequate knowledge, resources, effort and time. Death becomes contained by the specific medical explanation of its cause. Bauman's analysis of this tendency parallels Illich's thesis of iatrogenesis (1976) in which he suggests that the medical infiltration or medicalization of *all* aspects of everyday life have reduced our ability to deal with pain, suffering, and death. This infiltration has metamorphosed our concept of death from something that is a 'normal' part of life to something that is abnormal and unexpected, and which represents a failure of treatment. The second strategy that Bauman presents is the contemporary tendency to reify the 'here and now' and to minimize the concern with the past, or with the future.

While the medicalization and hospitalization of death spawned the wide-ranging, but abstract, theoretical and philosophical debate outlined above, a growing concern became visible from the 1950s about some of the specific *practical* and *experiential* consequences for individual patients, their families and companions and their professional carers. Such concern focused on isolation of dying people in hospital environments, on the dangers of new technologies that could blur the boundaries between living and dying, and on the difficulties faced by health care staff during the delivery of medical and nursing care to dying people together with the strategies employed to cope with repeated exposure to death. A new formulation of good death emerged from such work in which personal choice and 'awareness' of dying were central.

Various sources contributed to this reformulation: sociological analyses of the organization of care given to dying people (Glaser and Strauss 1965; Sudnow 1967); related studies looking at the education of nurses and the difficulties they experienced in caring for dying people; and the emergence of what has been termed the 'happy death' (Lofland 1978) or 'revival of death' (Walter 1994). Field's observation (1989) that 'open disclosure' of terminal prognoses has become an accepted, albeit ideal, aim of clinical practice within hospital areas has also been observed by other commentators (Armstrong 1984, 1987; Arney and Bergen 1984; Wouters 1990; Seale 1991b; May 1992a, b). It is suggested in these analyses that the development of hospice and palliative care has been particularly influential and persuasive in engendering such change. Essentially, what has been produced is a 'modern role' of dying in which the dying person and health care staff relate to one another in a well-defined way.

The work of Kübler-Ross (1969, 1975) promoted the idea that 'good death' was a matter of rejecting the institutionalization and 'deception' of dying people. She called for a return of death to the province of individual and familial control, and for a 'sharing of knowledge' (1970: 32) with dying people and their companions. Kübler-Ross suggested that in changing the approach to death, individuals would be enabled to embark on a journey of psychological preparation for their own death, or acceptance of the death of those close to them. She described 'stages' through which grief-stricken individuals move from denial to eventual acceptance. The concept of 'anticipatory grief' (Lindemann 1944; Murray Parkes 1970; Hampe 1975) has been central to work which has followed the lead of Kübler-Ross. Here, 'disclosure' and 'truth telling' (Armstrong 1987) are of central importance in facilitating the appropriate psycho-therapeutic adaptation of individuals to the threat of death and bereavement.

In Britain, the establishment of the hospice movement by Cicely Saunders was less overtly 'psycho-therapeutic', and more driven by humanitarian concerns to reduce the suffering of terminally ill people with intractable pain due to cancer. The establishment of St Christopher's Hospice was paralleled by pharmacological advances that made control of physical pain possible, and this allowed attention to turn to other dimensions of experience. Saunders's concept of 'total pain' encapsulated the philosophy developed during this period:

> . . . it soon became clear that each death was as individual as the life that preceded it and that the whole experience of that life was reflected in a patient's dying. This led to the concept of 'total pain' which was presented as a complex of physical, emotional, social and spiritual elements. The whole experience for a patient includes anxiety, depression, and fear; and concern for the family who will become bereaved; and often a need to find some meaning in the situation, some deeper reality in which to trust.
>
> (Saunders 1996: 1600)

As we saw in Chapter 1, this emphasis on the individuality of dying and of death, and the need for expression of feelings and of the development of a sense of meaning and of trust has been characterized as the cornerstone of 'post-modern' attitudes to good death. For example, Walter (1994: 56) refers to the contemporary 'expressive death' in which authority about the 'right' way to die has moved from the church or from the medical expert and is now vested solely in the dying individual. Such attitudes have taken hold in the broader field of health care and are exemplified by the emergence of palliative medicine as a distinct specialty. In nursing a general trend may be observed towards highlighting the emotional and psychological aspects of care and a reorganization of care delivery to enable a closer relationship between nurse and patient. Systems such as the nursing process and primary nursing exemplify such changes (Pearson 1988; Wright 1990; Manthey 1992).

May suggests that the generalized incorporation of the 'subjective' into health care has had the effect of creating an expectation of unproblematic dying. Here, individuals: '. . . die without pain, and are able to convey their feelings to near relatives and friends . . . having also resolved private fears and anxieties . . .' (May 1992a: 595). This scenario, however, contrasts sharply with the reality of dying for large swathes of the population. In high-technology areas of the hospital for example, patients can linger, without sensation of self, in a state of 'phenomenological death' (Kastenbaum 1969: 12) for hours, days and even weeks before 'biological death' ensues (Sudnow 1967). However, as Seale (1991c) and Field (1996) have highlighted in their detailed analyses, the more characteristic pattern of death in our society is that which creeps up slowly, and is interpreted not as a state of 'terminal illness' but as a natural part of the degeneration of ageing. In neither state are there dramatic moments of 'disclosure' or 'awareness', nor opportunities for self-determination. Further, specialist attention from highly trained 'death workers' who work to create the conditions in which good death can be achieved is not part of the experience of dying for the vast majority of people. 'Knowledge and control' (Field 1996: 256), the central features of the contemporary good death as 'concept' and as promoted actively by the hospice and palliative care movement, are conspicuously *absent* in death as concrete 'experience' but conspicuously *present* in terms of the popular expectations surrounding death.

By the end of the 1990s the concept of good death was generating more sustained critical commentary from sociologists. Hart *et al.* (1998) for example have agreed in their review of the subject that the predominance of good death ideologies can lead directly to the labelling of 'good' and 'bad' patients, and with it the exercise of normative control over the lives of dying people. In such a way the goals of the good death become unintentionally transmuted:

> Such goals at first thought appear both laudable and desirable. However, this exploration of the development of the good death concept exposes an ideology that constructs a socially approved form of dying and death with powerfully prescribed and normalized behaviours and choices.
>
> (Hart *et al.* 1998: 72)

These authors acknowledge also that significant challenges to this form of social control are emerging, for example through the pro-euthanasia movement. There is also evidence however that the good death ideology is being revised from within hospices themselves.

McNamara's studies of hospice care in Western Australia have led her to formulate the concept of the 'good enough' death (McNamara 1997). This, again, is an analysis which emphasizes the social factors which shape the experience of dying. It also draws on the argument, which we explore in more detail in the next chapter, that mainstream medicine and its associated technical imperatives constitute a threat to the principles of hospice care (McNamara *et al.* 1994, 1995). This analysis seeks to highlight conflicts between hospice ideals of the good death and organizational pressures centring around issues of cost-effectiveness, efficient administration and the routinization of care. It shows how in one Australian hospice, whilst nurses and other health professionals worked hard to maintain principles of the good death, there was growing acknowledgement that such an ideal could be difficult to sustain. 'Good' deaths were accompanied by awareness, acceptance and preparation, and a sense of peace and dignity. Conversely, the 'bad' death involved a lack of acceptance by the patient or family and a failure to engage with ideals of living life to the full to the very end. Faced with such tensions, McNamara suggests that hospice workers have come to embrace a more pragmatic and contingent notion of the 'good enough' death which gets as close as possible to the ideal, to the preferences of the deceased and which is consistent with the life the person had led (McNamara 1997).

We can see then that the hospice and palliative care movement has done a great deal to promote ideologies of the good death. At the same time it has become apparent that, even within the hospice environment, these are not always obtainable, hence the revisionism of the 'good enough' death. Beyond both of these points however lies the recognition that, for many, death continues to be far from 'good' or 'good enough'. In this sense many challenges to palliative care remain, in particular to move beyond the narrowness of focus which ultimately can only provide de-luxe dying for a minority (George and Sykes 1997).

The limits to palliation?

The future direction of palliative care development has recently become the subject of a wide-ranging debate. One key theme in this debate is the extent to which palliative care should retain its current specialist emphasis on the care of people with cancer. Saunders herself has suggested that her vision was more broadly based than has been subsequently interpreted: '... Terminal care should not be a facet of oncology, but of geriatric medicine, neurology, general practice and throughout medicine' (Saunders and Baines 1983: 2).

In spite of such aspirations, the exclusivity of the modern hospice movement has been expressed frequently as a cause for concern over the last 15–18 years (Hillier 1983; Wilkes 1984; O'Neill 1989; Seale 1989, 1991a; Clark 1994; Field 1994; James 1994). However, as James and Field (1992) have highlighted, this 'narrowness of focus' was also a key element in the success of the hospice movement. Tightly focused activity encouraged '. . . the development of highly specialised skills, techniques, and even technology, and [helped] generate the success vital to the continuity of the hospices' (James and Field 1992: 1367).

One of us, writing in 1993, noted that the success of palliative care in meeting the needs of people suffering from cancer has had its costs. In some senses, people dying with cancer are now relatively advantaged in terms of palliative care provision vis-à-vis those who die from other conditions. Further, in relation to hospice provision, there are '. . . general questions about the extent to which the hospice model is taking account of a range of social differences relating to age, gender, sexuality; family circumstances; religion and ethnicity' (Clark 1993c: 172).

Commentators both within and outside the specialty of palliative care are engaging increasingly in a debate about the extent to which it should widen its focus to include people with non-cancer disease; a group which constitutes the majority of those who die and who aspire increasingly to the powerful, culturally embedded meanings engendered by the 'good death' rhetoric. Thus Field, in an article about the emergence and role of palliative medicine as a specialty in its own right, has suggested that '. . . perhaps the "five star" care for the select few provided by hospice organisation should be replaced by "three star" care for all' (1994: 61).

Recently, Bosanquet (1997) has highlighted, from a health policy perspective, the great local variation in the availability of palliative care services for all seriously ill people and their informal carers. He points to the challenge of a projected 50 per cent increase in the need for palliative care services from people with non-cancer diagnoses (Higginson 1995), and to the increasing financial and structural pressures on palliative care. These latter pressures emanate from a competitive milieu which demands that service providers demonstrate cost-effectiveness, efficiency and evidence-based practice but which at the same time tends to act as a disincentive to coordination, cooperation and communication between different service providers. Such coordination is essential, argues Bosanquet, for the development of the local palliative care strategies recently called for (National Health Service Executive 1996), and may result both in significant improvements to the quality of life for dying people *and* in cost savings to health authorities. To support his argument Bosanquet draws on studies which have examined the benefits of introducing initiatives which encouraged district-wide coordination of cancer services (Raferty *et al.* 1996) or have explored the improvements that are possible in the role and development of primary care services in the delivery of palliative care (Eastaugh 1994; Robinson and Stacy 1994).

Bosanquet (1997) seems to suggest that palliative care can no longer rely on the sense of 'specialist mission' which has driven its development in the past and which, we would argue, has created perhaps a rather inward-looking and self-referential discipline. It may be that palliative care must instead look outwards and rise to the new challenges that have come from the heightening of awareness about the benefits of palliative care, its promise of the 'good death' and the widely based, but unequitably fulfilled, expectations of its availability:

> Palliative care has developed through a strong sense of specialist mission. It may well be difficult to share this mission with a wider audience, yet the gains in patients' quality of life would be great. Past investment in palliative care has created a valuable resource that is now local rather than exceptional, but there will be more pressure to demonstrate value for money. The challenge is how to use this resource so that all patients, including those with non cancer diagnoses, can benefit from access to better care. In an era of financial constraints, new alliances are needed for shared care if the full promise of palliative care is to be realised.
>
> (Bosanquet 1997: 1294)

Insofar then as hospice and palliative care has championed holism and the reform of the dominant health care system, it is now morally bound to engage in a critical debate about its future direction (Clark 1993c: 172–3).

George and Sykes (1997) give a valuable review of the range of special challenges presented to palliative care by a wide variety of non-cancer diseases. Our focus here, however, is the range of generic problems faced by the group of people who tend to suffer from the majority of such conditions: older people. We will examine, first, the special constraints with which the delivery of care in the community to this group is surrounded; and second, the empirical evidence available which gives insights into the problems of delivering palliative care to those dying from non-cancer disease within the acute hospital environment.

The experience of dying for older people: the disadvantaged majority?

People who die from chronic, degenerative, non-cancer disease tend to be aged over 65 years and to have a prolonged illness trajectory which culminates, in the majority of cases, in death within the confines of the acute hospital. In the UK, evidence has been accumulating since the early 1970s which suggests the experience of dying and death for this group of people and their carers is marked by extreme disadvantage in terms of palliative care provision. The most obvious indicator of this is the lack of deaths at home: the preferred place of death for most people (Hinton 1979; Wilkes 1984; Townsend et al. 1990).

Griffin (1991) reviewed several studies which explored why the majority of deaths occur in hospital and identified several factors which result in hospital admission:

- inability to control symptoms of disease, particularly pain;
- inadequate assessment of needs and planning for health care response;
- a lack of informal carers;
- a lack of support for informal carers.

The studies reviewed by Griffin (1991) were concerned with people of all ages who suffered from cancer, and the problems she identified were also found by Addington-Hall and McCarthy (1995) who conducted a retrospective interview-based survey of the family members of a nationally representative sample of people who died from cancer. Similar problems are experienced, but in a more acute form, by people who die from non-cancer disease. One of the earliest studies which drew attention to these difficulties was conducted by Cartwright *et al.* (1973) in a retrospective survey of a random sample of all deaths which had occurred over a one-year period in 40 areas of England and Wales. The aim here was to give a comprehensive picture of the way society cared for a predominantly old and sick group of people in the year before they died. The results of the study revealed a series of inadequacies in terms of service coverage, coordination and communication. There was, in particular, a lack of practical, social and emotional support for the relatives and friends who had cared for the people who had died. Domiciliary support such as home helps and district nurses was found to be sparse, and was conjoined with limited bed availability both in hospitals and in other institutions.

Seale and Cartwright (1994) went on to update this early study, examining the experience of dying among a random sample of people in ten areas by interviewing their relatives retrospectively. They found that people who died from cancer in the late 1980s were relatively advantaged in relation to those who died from non-cancer disease. This advantage was in terms both of the receipt of palliative care and informal support at home, and in terms of the coordination of services received in and out of hospital. Those who died from cancer were younger, had shorter periods of dependency, a greater number of relatives and friends available to care for them, and were able to take advantage of medical and nursing innovations that have tended to focus on the delivery of care to cancer patients. Those who died from non-cancer disease, by contrast, were older, tended to live alone with few sources of informal help, had a longer illness trajectory and received care that was comparatively poorly coordinated. This was particularly true of the relationship between hospital consultants and primary care services (Seale and Cartwright 1994).

A trend towards the gradual redefinition of 'health' need as 'social' need during the illnesses of old age and the erosion of state financial provision for the latter has recently come to awareness as possibly the fundamental barrier to the development of a palliative care approach in the management of life-threatening disease in older people. A recent report (Audit Commission

1997) has demonstrated that older people have suffered an unplanned, and almost accidental, fragmentation of their care and are currently the subjects of a 'vicious circle' in which they fall between the remits of responsibility of primary care, secondary care *and* social care. For example, NHS bed provision has fallen by 38 per cent since 1983, and the resulting gap in provision has been filled largely by independent, rather than local authority, residential and nursing home care. Numbers in private and voluntary homes have increased from 18,200 in 1983, to 148,500 in 1994 (Health Committee 1996). Black and Bowman (1997) have pointed out that the independent sector now provides the majority of long-term care for frail elderly people, but has tenuous links with statutory social and health services. One of the consequences of this, as Black and Bowman point out, is that '. . . the medical management of elderly people in community residential care remains poorly defined. It currently rests by default rather than design on the heavily burdened shoulders of general practitioners' (1997: 441). Further, standards of care are largely unmonitored in such homes and this, together with a lack of agreed minimum standards of care, encourages extreme variation in care conditions. Services provided by local authorities have clearly not developed to the same extent and indeed in some cases have been scaled down. The Audit Commission (1997) found evidence which shows, for example, that in 22 local authorities home help services have been reduced since 1993.

Rather than a health care context which encourages a palliative care approach to the health care needs of older people, the evidence reviewed suggests that a situation is developing which is inimical to the principles of palliative care. Older people who become ill experience a characteristic pattern of short admissions to hospital for 'acute' episodes of illness interspersed with long periods of time at home or in residential care receiving, in many cases, barely adequate attention from poorly coordinated, unregulated and over-stretched services. Palliative care needs in these circumstances tend to be neither recognized, assessed or planned for; at their most pressing and visible they are regarded as an 'acute' exacerbation of illness to be managed in the high-technology, increasingly hard-pressed confines of the hospital. From their perspective as specialists in geriatric medicine, Black and Bowman argue that the pressure placed on physicians to narrow their focus to acute services has aggravated this trend, encouraging a haphazard approach to community medical care and provoking idiosyncratic solutions ranging from naively planned community geriatrician posts to recruiting unaccountable visiting medical officers (Black and Bowman 1997: 441).

The personal meanings, experiences and costs which lie behind the broad trends outlined above can be illuminated forcefully by case study reports and by personal anecdote. We will refer to one recent example here, using the words of the stepson of a man who died in hospital following a prolonged period of severe chronic illness:

Jack . . . died in the end of a lung infection. But what in fact killed him was a combination of Parkinson's disease, severe arthritis, enlarged prostate and a damaged heart. During the year and a half of his final illness, he was treated by three different sets of specialists for these different ailments and was shunted back and forth between three different hospitals as each in turn was attended to. Communication between these hospitals was minimal. As a result, his notes were frequently lost or delayed or sent to the wrong hospital; he often spent days, even weeks without being treated at all, while the hospital he was in worked out what to do with him; and, most serious of all, he invariably lost out on the care of the ailments that weren't that particular hospital's speciality . . . The problem was that while there were lots of people in charge of different parts of Jack's body, no one was in charge of Jack, and therefore no one was able to determine which of his disorders should be prioritised and how the other symptoms should be dealt with . . . All of us in the family suspected that Jack was dying from the moment he contracted his first bladder infection to the day he finally did die a year and a half later . . . The fiction that, apart from the Parkinson's, his problems were temporary and that he would stride out of the hospital to resume a reasonably normal life was maintained to the end. It was a fiction that deprived Jack of the care he really needed.

(Hoyland 1997: 8–9)

The way in which health care delivery is currently structured is, it may be argued, at the root cause of such extreme suffering. The 'acute care culture' depends on a hospital organization structured around finding solutions to immediate, short-term health problems. This is done primarily by means of gathering a series of 'specialist' opinions each of which focuses on a particular aspect of 'the patient'. Decisions are then made on the basis of information that becomes progressively more narrow and less contextual in nature. Slomka (1992) has described the medical decision-making process as a 'cascade', in which there are a myriad of contributors, each of whom believes that their version of 'the patient' is the most cogent. Wendell-Moller (1996) has argued that the experience of dying is, in these circumstances, a 'roller coaster' in which

. . . attention is focused primarily on the management of physical symptoms. By focusing on the manageability of symptoms, the unmanageability of dying is superseded and deferred. As a result the process of dying is prolonged in such a way that it is often filled with uncertainty and ambivalence . . .

(Wendell-Moller 1996: 68)

Recently, empirical evidence has emerged which gives insights into the processes which constrain the delivery of palliative care within the acute hospital. In Chapter 8 we examine work which looks at palliative care delivery in UK hospitals. Here we will look at research from the United States. Treatment tends to be more 'aggressive' and interventionist in the US; however, we would argue that there are clear relevances for the situation in the UK given the acute focus of hospital care in this country and its apparent separation from primary health and social care. Local replication of research work conducted in the USA could yield invaluable information which is of direct relevance to the UK scene and which could form the basis for wider public and professional debate on these matters.

Dying in hospital: a complex challenge for palliative care

Ahronheim *et al.* (1996) conducted a retrospective chart-based review over a 13-month period of the care that two groups of elderly dying patients received in a large teaching hospital in the USA. The first group was constituted by 80 patients who were known to have been suffering from advanced dementia in the weeks and months preceding their death. This condition was marked by severe neurological incapacity and total dependence for all their physical needs. The other group was constituted by 84 patients who had been diagnosed as suffering from invasive metastatic cancer prior to death.

The review conducted by Ahronheim *et al.* indicated that although the majority of patients in both groups were designated as 'do-not-resuscitate' (DNR) (75 per cent of dementia patients and 82 per cent of cancer patients), many patients continued to receive invasive investigation and treatment until a few days before death. For example, in the dementia group 49 per cent of patients received 'invasive non-palliative' treatments such as haemodialysis, mechanical ventilation, enteral feeding and central venous cannulation. In the cancer group, 45 per cent of patients received such treatments. Further, the authors note that while an advance directive, which 31 per cent of cancer patients possessed compared to only 7.5 per cent of the dementia patients, did make invasive treatment less likely, it was not '. . . predictive of whether the patient received non-invasive diagnostic tests, invasive diagnostic tests, feeding tubes alone or a DNR order' (Ahronheim *et al.* 1996: 2096). An 'overwhelming' majority (88 per cent) of patients in this study received systemic antibiotics during their terminal period of hospital care. As Ahronheim *et al.* state in their conclusion, their study suggests that many incurably ill patients are given non-palliative interventions, and that palliative care may not even be considered as a possible option in the current cultural milieu of acute health care within the USA. Faber-Langendoen (1992, 1996) reported on a survey of deaths occurring in 'acute care beds' in four hospitals in Missouri over a two-year period. Her results support the key findings of Ahronheim *et al.*, and she publishes figures which demonstrate that 84 per cent of the patients who died in those hospitals had some intervention aimed at sustaining life in the period immediately before death. Further, she observes that interventions which were withdrawn from patients were done so in a piecemeal and inconsistent way. She reports, for example, that

> ... a large majority of patients, while having foregone some life sustaining treatment, continued to receive antibiotics and have laboratory blood tests performed within hours of death ...
>
> (Faber-Langendoen 1992: 2133)

While the work of Ahronheim *et al.* (1996) and Faber-Langendoen (1992, 1996) was retrospective, a major experimental, prospective and multi-site study has been conducted in the USA concerning similar issues. The title of the research is 'The Study to Understand Prognoses and Preferences for Outcomes and Risks of Treatment' (SUPPORT Project Principal Investigators 1995). This study, which started in 1989, had the stated aim of achieving a clearer understanding of the character of dying in American hospitals.

SUPPORT enrolled 9000 patients suffering from life-threatening illness in five hospitals over a four-year period. The first phase of the study was to describe in detail how hospitals care for patients who are at a very high risk of dying. Key findings from this phase were as follows:

- 80 per cent of those who died during phase one had a 'Do-not-resuscitate' order, but almost half of these orders were written within two days of death.
- 31 per cent of patients in phase one expressed a preference (to researchers) not to be resuscitated, but this was understood by slightly less than half of their lead clinicians.
- Of those patients who died in phase one, 38 per cent spent ten or more days in intensive care units.
- 50 per cent of all conscious patients who died in phase one were reported by their families as having moderate or severe pain.

The second phase of the study was the implementation and evaluation of an intervention aimed at resolving these problems highlighted in phase one. To this end, an intervention was designed which was aimed at improving communications between the relevant parties. First, the researchers provided doctors with brief written reports on their patients' probability of surviving up to six months, likelihood of being functionally impaired at two months and probability of surviving cardiopulmonary resuscitation. Second, doctors were provided with brief written reports regarding patients' views on life-sustaining treatment, presence of pain and desire for information. Third, specially trained nurse facilitators were given responsibility for initiating and maintaining communication between patients, their carers and their health care team.

Patients were randomized either to receive the intervention or to continue with the usual medical care. Data pertaining to the key issues highlighted in phase one were then gathered from the two groups and the results compared. The results indicated that there was no significant difference between the two groups regarding the four key issues: the timing of do-not-resuscitate orders remained the same; patient–physician communication did not improve; reported pain levels remained static; and high levels of technology attended a significant proportion of deaths.

In a detailed analysis of the results of the SUPPORT study, commentators contributing to a special supplement of the Hastings' Center Report (1995) identified a range of possible factors which underpin the characteristics of modern hospital care for dying people. For example, Lo (1995) suggests that the SUPPORT intervention did not address the wider organizational and cultural issues in which the autonomy and accountability of individual physicians remains central to the process of care decision making. These factors encourage physicians to rely on judgements informed by their own expertise rather than on judgements made by others (such as nurses), since they may be perceived as less accountable for patient care. Thus a narrow, biomedical interpretation of prognosis and 'quality of life' is encouraged; an interpretation that may neither correspond to perspectives held by nurses, families or primary care staff, nor allow an incorporation of those perspectives into an evaluation of what constitutes an 'appropriate' course of action.

The Hastings' Center Commentary further points out that in the SUPPORT study, many patients seemed to want high-technology interventions, saying that they feared these less than the perceived risk that clinicians might give up hope of cure prematurely. According to personal values, then, some patients may want interventions that other people regard as inappropriately aggressive. Lo (1995) suggests that patients are often overly optimistic about their prognoses and that this, together with the poor disclosure of information to patients, is the root cause of the demand for continuation of aggressive treatment. He suggests that patients are more likely to decline such interventions following detailed and repeated discussions with their physicians:

> ... in our experience almost all disagreements between physicians and patients or families over the appropriateness of life sustaining interventions can be resolved after repeated discussions. These discussions may be difficult and time consuming, requiring several hours a day ... over a period of weeks ...
>
> (Lo 1995: S.8)

Despite the successes of its expansion and diversification, it should also be clear from the foregoing discussion that the transitions from terminal, to hospice and to palliative care have also been beset with tensions and difficulties. Many of these revolve around definitions, models and protocols for palliative care; and here we see shifting sands with much debate and a variety of viewpoints. There is a great deal more to the definition of palliative care than a cursory reference to its Latin roots and to the World Health Organisation's statement of 1990. We hope in this chapter to have shed some light on this. Likewise we have shown how the concept of the good death, which is so closely tied to hospice and palliative care philosophy, needs to be appraised in the light of its historical origins, but also in relation to current empirical evidence about how it is being constructed in specialist palliative care settings. Finally, we have emphasized that within the current mode of operation adopted by palliative care, with its emphasis on cancer and care in specialist units, a huge unfinished agenda remains. The experience of palliative care still characterizes a minority of deaths around the world; how palliative care for all can be achieved remains a major object of concern.

The somewhat pessimistic conclusions of the Hastings' Center Special Supplement are captured in the words of Annas:

> . . . in the high-tech, high pressure environment [of the hospital] there is little room for thoughtfulness, for the intrusion of human values, or for conversation with the patient or family. The primary values are action and technology oriented; the imperative is to use all available medical technologies for the patient or for practice . . . add cost pressures to treat more patients more quickly, and the care of the dying in hospitals is likely to get worse, not better.
>
> (Annas 1995: S.12)

The widespread use of palliative care terminology and the currency of the 'good death' as an ideal has shown the extent to which hospice and palliative care is regarded as an integral feature of the service which should be delivered to all dying people. However, as shown in this chapter, hospice and palliative care faces many challenges if it is to adapt to the vast areas of need that exist beyond its traditional remit of cancer care. A fundamental challenge is the resolution of the tension between the legacy of independence, innovation, and demedicalization and the risks posed to those values by collaboration and integration with mainstream, medically dominated, health care. Our next chapter turns to a close examination of these issues.

6 Routinization and medicalization

Thirty years after the emergence of the modern hospice movement and ten years after the establishment of palliative care as a medical specialty, concerns are being expressed about the possible subversion of the founding principles of hospice and palliative care. Two critical debates may be discerned in the literature. The first is related to the Weberian thesis that social movements are subject to an inevitable process of historical and social change and must evolve eventually into inflexible, professionalized, rule-bound, bureaucratic institutions. Commentators who adhere to this 'routinization' argument express particular anxieties about the vulnerability of small, previously independent hospices to wider institutional influence and control, whether within the hospice and palliative care movement *or* within mainstream health care. The second debate, which is tightly linked to the first, concerns the argument that contemporary hospice and palliative care is becoming increasingly medicalized, partly as a result of reincorporation into mainstream health care, but also, more insidiously, as a result of the apparent willingness of the hospice and palliative care movement to be drawn into the pervasive development of a form of 'therapeutic' culture in which the universal experience of suffering is brought into the remit of professional health care and recharacterized as a 'problem' with a medical solution. In this chapter we address each of these issues in turn and also explore their interrelationships.

The 'routinization' thesis

It was as early as 1986 that Emily Abel first put forward the notion, using the example of the American hospice movement, that some form of institutionalization might be taking place with the effect of curbing hospice innovation (Abel 1986). Often overlooked in the subsequent 'routinization' debate, her paper merits further consideration. Abel argues that hospices in the USA had the 'revolutionary' mission of transforming the American health care system. There were several elements to this programme. The hospices sought to minimize the control of physicians, to place more equal value on the skills of diverse professionals and to bridge the gap between expert and non-expert. Within the hospices death was to be seen as a 'natural event' rather than a technological failure, and the family was to be the unit of care. Finally, there would be a particular emphasis on home care, itself a major challenge to the institutional and bureaucratic character of modern health care. As we saw in Chapter 4, the American hospices grew rapidly and took various forms: home health programmes, as well as some free-standing in-patient units and services allied to hospitals. Despite being divorced from the mainstream and a relative indifference to fund-raising issues and financial worries, American hospices, for Abel, quickly found themselves drawn into the predominant health care system. This brought practical and administrative advantages, assisted in spreading the hospice message and led to inclusion in Medicare and wider programmes of accreditation, licensure and certification. At the same time it appeared to jeopardize hospice identity. Abel concludes that the American hospices proved *both* progressive and conservative. They achieved the former by a rejection of prevailing values within the medical establishment, but they demonstrated the latter through an emphasis on individual solutions, familistic values and charitable principles. For Abel then the hospice movement is seen as a counter-institution which, paradoxically, has survived through incorporation into the mainstream.

The most detailed application of the routinization thesis as it relates to hospices was put forward by James and Field in 1992. They argue that while the post-Second World War social climate created certain preconditions in which the hospice movement could take root and flourish, it was the powerfully influential leadership of Cicely Saunders that acted as a 'catalyst' for social change. James and Field use Weber's concept of 'charisma' to examine Cicely Saunders's leadership, focusing on Weber's view that the charisma of exceptional individuals is 'the agency which produces radical innovation in institutions and established beliefs' (James and Field 1992: 1365). However, this is an agency that is inherently unstable because of a dependence upon non-institutionally sanctioned power, creative energy, and irregular financial support. Such leadership, according to Weber, can only resist reincorporation into the wider value system for as long as the number of followers remains small and the development of 'rational' administrative bureaucracy can be avoided. History, for Weber, thus 'alternates between charisma and routinization through bureaucracy . . .' (1992: 1365).

James and Field (1992: 1367) note that the success of the modern hospice movement depended upon a '. . . singleness of vision, an intensity of purpose and a narrowness of focus', and so identify four elements of charismatic leadership that were integral to its development:

- the role of Cicely Saunders as a highly visible leader;
- the spiritual 'calling' which inspired many to become involved with hospices;
- the hospice vision of terminal care with its narrowness of focus;
- the oppositional stance of the movement to mainstream health care.

As James and Field point out, 'charisma' made up of these elements resonated with wider public attitudes towards, and concern about, care for dying people. This public resonance engendered, in part, the huge trend in charitable donations, voluntary involvement (both individual and organizational) *and* the interest of mainstream health care professionals in hospice-style care giving to dying people. Further, it encouraged the detailed cultural specification of the elements constituting a dignified and peaceful 'good death'. In this way, the hospice movement became absorbed gradually into the national psyche and incorporated into the fabric of its wider public institutions; we comment further on this in Chapter 7. James and Field note (1992: 1368) that the cancer charities of Macmillan Cancer Relief and the Marie Curie Foundation were particularly influential in shaping the development and focus of the hospice movement; and that, further, hospice care became a symbol within mainstream health care of good practice with dying people, leading to a huge demand for education, research and a dissemination of hospice-style care to non-cancer patients.

The thrust of James and Field's argument is that all of these perhaps *unintended* developments and demands have had far-reaching effects upon the character of the hospice movement, causing it to metamorphose into a large bureaucracy. They draw on the work of Andreski (1984), suggesting that the modern hospice movement now shares some of the following features of ideal-typical bureaucratic institutions:

- the strict division of spheres of authority determined by general rules, laws and regulations;
- a hierarchy of offices and the channelling of communication through proper hierarchical channels (i.e. a strict division of labour);
- the training of official post holders;
- a separation of official activities from private affairs;
- duties discharged in accordance with rules.

James and Field argue that these features of organizational development have been paralleled by the reprofessionalization of terminal care; a trend towards the quantitative style of evaluation and audit of the 'quality' of hospice care; and an emergent dependence upon health authorities for financial support. New tensions and conflicts have been created which militate against hospice ideals:

> There is a danger of goal displacement, with the core goal of effective, humane care of dying people is [sic] in danger of being partially displaced by other activities which were initially subsidiary to this goal. We have already indicated the pressure from clinical/medical audit and the 're-professionalization' of hospice care upon the practice of holistic care – a displacement of focus and practice back towards the more traditional medical conceptions of disease and its treatment, to the possible detriment of other 'softer' aspects of care. Other factors are the diversification of hospice activities; the increasingly important role of educational activities; staffing changes which mean that second, third, fourth, fifth and sixth generation staff are unlikely to have the drive and commitment of the pioneer staff; and potential pressures to accept non cancer patients.
>
> (1992: 1372)

Since the publication of James and Field's rather pessimistic characterization of the contemporary hospice movement, other authors have directed their attention to key aspects of their thesis. Below we will examine in some detail the 'medicalization' aspects of their argument, drawing on recent work of social theorists who have developed the concept of medicalization to include more than just a concern with the extent to which hospice and palliative care has re-embraced the use of invasive treatments and physical treatments. Before doing this however, we examine recent developments in the argument that the current generation of hospice staff is poorly equipped to enact hospice ideals because of a lack of commitment to the spiritual and religious aspects of the vocational 'calling' associated with hospice care. At the end of the chapter the empirical evidence which supports or refutes the routinization and medicalization theses will be examined.

Spirituality and hospice care

Bradshaw (1996) examined the 'routinization' thesis in terms of Weber's claim that the secularization of society has led to the replacement of religious vocation by the 'iron cage' of duty. Bradshaw defines secularization in the modern sociological sense as 'the widespread decline in religious traditions as their beliefs and values no longer hold popular respect' (1996: 409), but points out that it is only in the twentieth century that 'secular' has come to mean separation from the spatial jurisdiction of the church and, more fundamentally, from the Christian conscience. As Bradshaw notes, during medieval times 'secular' was a term used to describe clergy who practised in the community rather than within the physical confines of a church or to describe concern with the present life, rather than with life after death. The example of Florence Nightingale's conception of nursing is used by Bradshaw to underline the difference between the modern-day and medieval meanings of secular:

> ... it is helpful to appreciate that the nineteenth century secularisation of nursing pioneered by Nightingale was different. For Nightingale it was more akin to the medieval idea, a movement away from the religious order and religious profession ... into a lay profession. The religious foundation and inspiration remained. Nursing was maintained as a spiritual vocation.
>
> (Bradshaw 1996: 410)

Bradshaw goes on to highlight the many parallels between the emergence of nursing and the emergence of palliative and hospice care, arguing that the latter is the 'quintessential' place of nursing where 'care' is at its most fundamental. She draws particularly on the early writings of Cicely Saunders to demonstrate the Christian calling behind Saunders's efforts in establishing the hospice movement. However, she argues that the subsequent development of both nursing and hospice care and their contemporary emphasis on professionalization has undermined the Christian ethic of care. 'Care' in the professionalized 'rational' world of modern nursing and hospice care becomes a routinized and secularized attempt to facilitate the behavioural expression of 'good death' (cf McNamara *et al.* 1994) in which the *process* of dying is more important than the moment of death itself. The role of hospice care and of nursing as a 'spiritual anchor' (Bradshaw 1996: 410) for those who are dying becomes marginalized, and 'real love' is replaced by the 'self conscious application of psychosocial skills and techniques' (1996: 412). Compassion and meaning, in this argument, are replaced by a spiritually empty exercise in expertise in which, Bradshaw maintains, there is a 'positive risk of manipulation' (1996: 414) due to the unevenness of the relationship between the ill person and his or her 'expert' caregiver. Bradshaw goes so far as to argue that an earlier 'universal' moral pattern of society, captured in the religious spirituality of the early modern hospice movement and its emphasis on compassion, has given way to values which 'rest in whatever means and techniques produce psychological effectiveness' (1996: 413). For Bradshaw, the emphasis on the acquisition of psychosocial skills and knowledge not only devalues the importance of 'moral quality' and compassion in professional care giving, but also obscures the 'genuine' source of truth, morality and compassion: theological grounding. Bradshaw argues that without religious values in hospice work, '... reality is meaningless: an empty future without hope. Death is the inevitable end that cuts off all hope' (1996: 417).

Bradshaw's argument that 'genuine' compassion and morality stem from religious values can be criticized on several grounds. First, we may question the necessary association that she implies between a vocational sense of 'calling' and religious values. Vocation may have various foundations, and altruism and a desire to serve one's fellows may not necessarily be based in religious conviction. Further, in her emphasis on Christianity, the cross-cultural dimension of hospice development is ignored. It is both ethnocentric and inaccurate to imply that Christian values are the best foundation for an ethic of care. Recent analyses of the international development of hospice and palliative care (Clark *et al.* 1997a; Saunders and Kastenbaum 1997) demonstrate amply the huge variety of cultural and religious values that may underpin care and compassion within the hospice and palliative care movement. Similarly, her argument that an emphasis on professionalization of hospice and nursing care is somehow detrimental to the more fundamental intuitive skills of 'real love' must be examined critically. Walter (1997a) subjects the issue of spirituality in hospice and palliative care to critical scrutiny, examining first, the possible meanings of 'spiritual care', and second, the argument that the professionalization of spiritual care is another manifestation of routinization. We review his arguments here to try to widen the debate beyond Bradshaw's polemic.

Walter identifies three possible solutions to the delivery of 'spiritual care' to dying people within a 'fundamentally secular, rational and this worldly context' (1997a: 22). First, as Bradshaw has argued, spirituality can be narrowly confined as the proper concern only of religious members of staff within small hospices. As Walter and Bradshaw both point out, this may lead to tensions and conflict as the organization expands and has to look 'outside' to secular staff to fulfil its duty of professional care to ill people. Walter describes how secular staff may feel that 'spiritual care' is an infringement of privacy, while religious staff may feel that a charismatic 'gift of discernment', which endows a special ability to know when someone needs spiritual comfort, is most widely available among those within their 'own' group. As Walter points out, the idea that spiritual care depends on a 'God given' gift throws up major problems not only for the care of dying *outside* the hospice movement but also within the large bureaucracies of which contemporary hospices may be, or become, a part:

> ... how is this gift, this charisma, to be routinized in the larger and more bureaucratic institutions that hospices may turn into, or in the large hospitals that hospices aim to influence? Can thousands be expected to have this gift? If not, can such a gift be taught? If all nurses are expected to provide spiritual care, how may those without this particular gift or indeed without religious commitment discern when a patient is raising spiritual issues and know how to respond?
>
> (Walter 1997a: 24)

Walter argues that the most straightforward solution to such problems is to locate spiritual care firmly within the specialist remit of the clergy, and to assume that

- spiritual is the same as religious;
- only some people are religious;
- non-religious and non-ordained staff are not competent to deal with spiritual needs.

This group of assumptions allows professional staff to get on with the business of delivering clinical and social care, and even emotional care, but leaves the 'tricky business' (1997a: 24) of spiritual care to others. However, as Walter points out, the major problem with such a conception is that it does not 'fit' with the concept of holistic care which, as we have seen in the previous chapter, underpins the most basic premise of hospice and palliative care. Further, in a more narrow sense, it implies that only some dying people have spiritual needs and that 'ordinary' staff cannot help them with these needs. The third conception of spiritual care identified by Walter seems to reassociate 'spiritual' with 'holistic' and does not depend upon a narrow identification with the religious conviction either of the patient or staff member. Walter traces the emergence of a new meaning of spiritual care within British and North American literature:

> This identifies the spiritual with the search for meaning and has more to do with human spirit as the animating or vital principle in a person – 'the breath of life' – than with religion, narrowly defined . . . although only a minority of patients may have explicitly religious concerns in the churchy sense of the word, a majority have existential concerns of a wider nature.
>
> (Walter 1997a: 25)

Walter argues that Cicely Saunders has been particularly influential in propagating and encouraging this particular formulation of 'spiritual', basing her understanding on logotherapy: the therapy of meaning. Writing recently, Saunders has indeed made clear her commitment to responding to universally 'human' concerns of the 'inner' self and relationship to others, rather than to selectively 'religious' concerns and the relationship only to God (Saunders 1996). Indeed, a close reading of Cicely Saunders's early writings (Clark 1998b) shows how her preoccupations were with the interrelationships between physical, social, psychological and spiritual problems. Moreover she sought to address these in non-Christians (David Tasma himself, her first terminal care patient, was a Jew) and non-believers (the first patient she ever described in a publication had been 'a preacher of atheism' at London's Hyde Park Corner; Saunders 1958: 37). So despite the overtly Christian language of Cicely Saunders's writings at this time, we should not be led into thinking that there was any sense of exclusivity about her position on matters of religion. Indeed, it is perhaps a strength of her concept of 'total pain' (Clark 1998c) that by combining the physical, social, psychological and spiritual, it can be developed and utilized across the range of cultural settings.

Far from Bradshaw's argument that Christianity and religious conviction is a necessary and fundamental aspect of the ability to relate in a 'genuinely' spiritual and non-exploitative sense to others, it would seem that Saunders herself, although personally a Christian, has not seen a necessary or exclusive relationship between religiosity and spiritual care. The ability to relate to others, to listen and to be 'with' those who face death were seen as perhaps more important in the context of a 'real' world where religious conviction is only part of the richness of human life and of suffering. Saunders's (1988) description of what she called 'spiritual pain' is used by Walter in an earlier publication (1994: 102) to highlight the similarities between her conception of spiritual care and wider notions of compassionate, skilled nursing care:

> We can always persevere with the practical. Care for the physical needs, the time taken to elucidate a symptom, the quiet acceptance of a family's angry demands, the way nursing care is given, can carry it all and can reach the most hidden places. This may be all we can offer to inarticulate spiritual pain – it may be well enough as our patients finally face the truth on the other side of death.
>
> (Saunders 1988, quoted in Walter 1994: 102)

Saunders's implicit parallel between 'total patient care' and the relief of spiritual distress has been widely accepted within the nursing profession. As Savage (1995) notes, caring 'for' in a practical, task-oriented sense has been replaced in nursing discourse by the language of caring 'about' in an emotional, private and person-centred sense; and a new emphasis is placed on the quality of the interpersonal relationship between nurse and patient. The widespread reorganization of nursing to allow allocation of 'named' or 'primary' nurses to each patient may be seen as reflecting these concerns, as well as attempts to institutionalize opportunities for personalized exchanges of the type so vividly described by Saunders. It might be argued that the professionalization of nursing has resulted in the enhancement and wholehearted pursuit of the 'holistic' values associated with palliative care, making the experience of dying more bearable and meaningful for people in many settings of care. Indeed, much of the recent literature concerning the professionalization of nursing is concerned to re-establish such values at the very centre of clinical practice, research and education (Pincombe *et al.* 1996; Engebretson 1997; Raudonis and Acton 1997). Professionalization and compassion in this literature are portrayed 'hand in hand' rather than 'back to back'. However, some commentators on the professionalization of compassion in nursing and in palliative care take Bradshaw's line, and use aspects of the 'routinization' thesis to argue that the growing incorporation of the 'subjective' in nursing is merely another indicator of the growing fragility, indeed artificiality, of 'meaningful' human relationships between professional and patient. Forming relationships that meet the demands inherent within the discourse of holism is seen as fraught with difficulty and hidebound by organizational forces outside individual influence, beyond an individual understanding of their 'true' nature. Essentially, professional–patient relationships are understood as unequal, transitory and subject to shifting and contradictory institutional pressures in which 'holism' is not highly prized. James and Field (1996) point to the web of structural constraints impinging on nurses' work, such as financial limits, pressures of cross-disciplinary working and divisions between health and social care. They argue that social structural and organizational constraints may render nurses effectively powerless to pursue the 'holism' on which palliative care depends:

> ... [t]he delivery of care by nurses to dying people is a constant and perhaps increasingly difficult battle to overcome the limitations of the health structures within which such care is given ... pressures within the NHS may be leading away from the possibility of providing the 'total' care of the 'whole' person which is such a vital part of the good nursing care of dying people ...
>
> (James and Field 1996: 79)

More fundamentally, Walter echoes Bradshaw's concerns when he notes that the institutionalization of Cicely Saunders's widely based conception of spiritual care as an integral part of all 'holistic' care may involve a process of 'normalization' in which spiritual and existential concerns are converted into the 'discourse of clients, needs, goals, care plans and outcomes' (1997: 27). The individual approach so clearly portrayed in Saunders's writings may then be lost in a 'routinization' and rationalization of 'therapy speak' in which patient and carer are locked into a stylized relationship framed by expected behaviours.

The acquisition of 'counselling' techniques in nursing, the pervasive and uncritical embrace of 'total patient care' and the popular idea that 'good death' involves movement through certain defined 'stages' have all been cited as evidence of an exercise, albeit in an essentially unconscious manner, of a routinized and insidious form of social control. Lupton (1995), for example, has examined critically the role of nurses in the clinical encounter. Lupton suggests that the 'new holism' of nursing, which demands the attainment of intimacy between nurse and patient, is a manifestation of a wider 'clinical gaze' exercised by medicine:

> The current focus in nursing on 'knowing' and understanding patients, to the extent of gauging their emotional states and the nature of their relationships with family members, may be viewed as an even greater extension of medical surveillance into the lives of patients. To incite patients to speak, to allow their voices to be heard, may render them more vulnerable to the exercise of disciplinary, and possibly coercive, power than if they remain silent.
>
> (Lupton 1995: 161)

Lupton's characterization of holistic nursing care as a form of surveillance is a recent development of a long-established critical perspective in social theory: that of 'medicalization'. This perspective emerged in various forms as a critical commentary on the post-Second World War professional dominance of medicine. As indicated above, James and Field (1992) identified the existence of this commentary as one of a range of social and intellectual trends which allowed the hospice movement to flourish. An important aspect of their thesis of routinization concerns the extent to which the contemporary hospice movement is apparently being reincorporated into the institutional and professional jurisdiction of mainstream medical care. The emergence of palliative medicine as a specialty in 1987 is cited as evidence of the latter, with anxieties expressed that this may signal a wholesale re-embracing of the biomedical model of care and the professional hegemony of medicine at the expense of the principles of holism (James and Field 1992; Biswas 1993; Field 1994). The risk that 'medicalization' may jeopardize any special identity that palliative care has developed is usually seen in terms of its institutional affiliation. In its broadest sense however medicalization refers to a *manner of thinking* about sickness, health, death and dying which is all-embracing, and from which hospice and palliative care have no special immunity.

The medicalization thesis

The literal meaning of to 'medicalize' simply means to 'make medical' and the emergence of medical ways of thinking has been linked in popular thought to a socially progressive growth of rationality and humanitarianism. The critical influence of medicine on post-war society was recognized as an important area of study by sociologists, who began to draw attention to the *socially constructed*, rather than *biologically given*, aspects of health, illness and disease. Talcott Parsons, working as a sociologist in the United States during the 1950s, was centrally concerned with the way in which the institution of medicine contributed to the overall smooth operation of society by the containment of 'deviant' states of health. He introduced the concept of the 'sick role' in which doctor and patient relate to one another in clearly defined ways which ensure that 'illness' does not disrupt normal social life. Each has particular rights and duties which are acted out in a reciprocal spirit of tacit agreement. However, later theorists took a more critical stance, associating the social control functions of medicine with the disempowerment of individuals, with an increasing tendency to define 'normal' aspects of life as medical problems, and with the advancement of medicine as a form of pervasive, and in some ways invisible, ideological control. Writing during the 1970s, Freidson, for example, observed how

As late as the nineteenth century, medicine was a relatively unimport-
ant institution, humble before the majesty of religion and the law. But,
with the growth of medical science, more and more human behaviour
began to stem from specific 'causes' over which prayer, human choice
and will had little control . . . from this core of scientific discovery
grew a vague halo of authority that encouraged the wholesale definition
of medical definitions of deviance into areas of behaviour previously
managed by religion and the law . . .

(Freidson 1970: 248)

Freidson clarified his argument by reference to the work of Szasz (1964),
who was concerned primarily with the growth of psychiatry. Szasz noted
how 'illness' has come to define not only manifestations of structural or
functional disorders of the physical body, but also disability and suffering emanating from *mental* states such as depression, anxiety and neur-
osis. For Szasz, 'sickness' was a misnomer for 'problems of living'. He
argued that these are properly located within the moral, socio-cultural and
political spheres and cannot be regarded as neutral states of being that can
only be explained by 'objective' science. Szasz's stance is one example of a
wide-ranging critique, known as the 'anti-psychiatry' movement, which
argued that the way in which post-war society used medical *labels* to manage 'deviance' effectively neutralized political threats from non-conformist
individuals:

. . . psychiatrists began to call illness . . . anything and everything in
which they could detect any sign of malfunctioning, based on no matter what norm. Hence agoraphobia is an illness because no one should
be afraid of open spaces. Homosexuality is an illness because hetero-
sexuality is the social norm. Divorce is an illness because it signals the
failure of marriage . . .

(Szasz 1964: 44–5)

The recognition that the attribution of a 'sickness' label is a social process
spawned a number of theorizations which attempted to explain the ways
in which an individual's social identity and sense of self are developed. The
writings of Erving Goffman (1963, 1968) were perhaps among the most
influential of these, suggesting the intricate processes whereby certain individuals, or groups of individuals, are stigmatized, segregated and stripped
of their individuality during the attribution and treatment of 'sickness'. A
further highly influential school of social enquiry combined the insights of
Parsons, Freidson and interactionist theorists such as Goffman to examine
the various ways in which medical 'dominance' is achieved during everyday
interaction between doctor and patient (Bloor 1977; Strong 1979; Silverman
1987). Indeed, much of the work of medical sociologists in the recent past
has concerned this issue and has led to a huge body of empirical studies

which suggest that the medical encounter is a means of perpetuating the hegemony of medicine by the exclusion of 'lay' explanations and definitions of illness and of the lived experience of illness. Kleinman's work (1988) detailing the experience of chronic illness from the patient's perspective is only one of a number of studies which have highlighted the dissonance between the subjective experience of 'illness' and the medical concern with an apparently 'objective' bodily state which doctors describe as 'disease'.

Glaser and Strauss's (1965) study of the way in which dying was concealed as a diagnosis in American hospitals was one of a number of enquiries which employed insights informed by the medicalization thesis. A central concern of these studies was to explain how the socially disruptive threats of dying and death were managed during social interaction.

Glaser and Strauss described the interactions between staff and patients in six hospitals in San Francisco. They introduced the concept of 'awareness': 'Who, in the dying situation, knows what about the probabilities of death for the dying patient' (1965: ix). The primary focus of their analysis was on the types of social action engaged by health care staff to avoid direct disclosure of a poor prognosis and how this led to the isolation of dying persons and those close to them. Sudnow's 1967 study was similarly concerned with the types of social action with which dying people are surrounded in modern medical environments. He argued that death and dying in hospitals is interpreted in such a way that 'social' death practices precede bodily death. For example Sudnow described how the bodies of still living, but comatose, patients would be partially prepared for the morgue or removed from the main ward areas. Building on the early work of Glaser and Strauss (1965) and Sudnow (1967), Quint (1967) (latterly Benoliel-Quint (1977)) highlighted the lack of education given to nurses about how to care for dying patients in hospitals. Benoliel-Quint argued that this demonstrated both the low status of caring work, and a societal rejection of care of dying as an important issue. Benoliel-Quint described how nurses must attend to the intimate needs of dying patients within a depersonalized environment predicated on the denial of death and the procuration of cure. Later studies, using similar methodologies, have replicated some of these findings. For example, Field (1989) showed that while attitudes to disclosure of terminal prognoses have changed, the organization of nursing work in some settings still encourages pretence and a routinization of care giving. Robbins (1998) compares two studies of communication between clinical staff and patients, one which took place in hospital (Peräkylä 1989) and the other in the community (Hunt 1991). Both authors identified a range of 'frames' or 'roles' used by staff in dealing with death and dying. Thus, sometimes a task-oriented frame would be applied at the expense of other more social or 'person'-centred frames. Robbins (1998) suggests that such 'frames' can be regarded as strategies used by staff to manage the daily stresses of caring for dying people.

Writers who focus on the clinical encounter between doctors, nurses and their patients have been criticized for taking inadequate account of the wider social and economic context within which such exchanges take place. In describing what is known as the 'political economy' perspective on medicalization Gerhardt (1989: 269–73) draws on the work of Zola (1972, 1975), Conrad (1975, 1979) and McKeown (1965) who focused on the role of medicine as a repository of state control in which medical science is used to support the interests of elite social groupings rather than those of the population as a whole.

One highly original and extremely influential author taking this stance has been Ivan Illich (1976) who wrote a polemic in which he attributed widespread 'iatrogenic' sickness (i.e. that resulting from a generalized societal dependency on medical intervention) to the dominance of medicine itself. For Illich, *social* iatrogenesis results when

> . . . health care is turned into a standardised item, a staple, when all suffering is hospitalised and homes become inhospitable to birth, sickness and death . . . or when suffering, mourning and healing outside the patient role are labelled a form of deviance . . .
>
> (Illich 1976: 49)

Illich argues that an insidious culture of dependence results from this transformation of the social management of 'sickness', arguing that this constitutes another form of iatrogenesis: *cultural* iatrogenesis. This he described as a state in which

> . . . medically sponsored behaviour and delusions restrict the vital autonomy of people by undermining their competence in growing up, caring for each other, and ageing, or when medical intervention cripples personal responses to pain, disability, impairment, anguish and death . . .
>
> (Illich 1976: 271)

Echoing the central argument of the routinization debate, Illich argues that it is industrialization and economic growth which have given rise to iatrogenic sickness, since these processes have encouraged the growth of professional bureaucracies which stand to intervene between the individual and his/her environment. Illich echoes the work of Szasz and of Parsons in his argument that 'sickness' is subject to historical and cultural specification, and to a societal 'need' to contain potentially subversive deviance. This recognition of the *historical* contingency of sickness definitions has been most highly developed in the work of Foucault (1973, 1977). Foucault offers a theorization of medicalization based on an analysis of the inter-relationship between 'disciplinary' power, clinical practice, and the private lives and beliefs of individuals. He suggests that in the modern period, medical ideas and knowledge constitute a 'discourse', or coherent system of knowledge and action, within which all aspects of health, illness, disease and bodily experience are defined and brought under disciplinary control. This is a control which is disseminated beyond identifiable social groups such as medical practitioners, becoming instead incorporated into social life as a whole. The widespread popularity of 'fitness' and 'dietary' monitoring and the increasing popular concern with the pre-emption of physical and psychological disease might be seen as evidence of the overarching persuasion and ideological control of medical ways of thinking. Foucault argues that in contemporary society, medicine has become a form of panoptical 'gaze' internalized and exercised by private individuals and constraining the ways in which we all think. He argues that medicine frames the way in which we think about our lives *and* our deaths:

> ... this positive medicine ... marked the beginning of that fundamental relation that binds man to his original finitude ... health replaces salvation ... health offers modern man the obstinate and yet reassuring face of his finitude; in it death is endlessly repeated but is also exorcised ... this relation of man to death authorises a scientific discourse in a rational form and opens up a source of language that unfolds endlessly in the void left by the absence of the gods ...
>
> (Foucault 1973: 197–8)

Bauman (1992) builds on this to argue that the medicalization theory most helpfully explains the current preoccupation with the individual causes of death and their avoidance by careful bodily monitoring. Following a similar argument to Ariès (1981), he argues that death, through the forces of medicalization, becomes a 'problem' of professional health care, rather than an accepted, inevitable and visible fact of life to be dealt with in the family and community and by means of spiritual preparation:

> ... death ... is held out of the agenda, elbowed out by another truth: that each particular cause of death (most importantly death which threatens the particular person, me at the particular moment, now) can be resisted, postponed, or avoided altogether. Death as such is inevitable, but each concrete instance of death is contingent ... all deaths have causes ... We do not hear of anyone dying of mortality. They die only of causes ... I can do anything to defy mortality ...
>
> (Bauman 1992: 5–6)

Foucault's conception of medicalization centres around the idea that the power of medicine is all-embracing, its popular appeal seductive, and, as Lupton (1997: 98) notes, '... productive rather than merely confining'. For Foucault, medical ways of thinking actively produce the ways in which we *understand, experience* and *self-regulate* our bodies. Medical power, in this perspective, does not belong to particular elite groups at the expense of the powerlessness of weaker groups; rather it exists in the relations between social groupings and is dispersed within widely accepted notions of what properly constitutes 'good health', 'good death' and bodily and psychological 'fitness'.

Foucault's arguments have been used by some commentators to suggest that the trend towards the development of 'holism' in medical practice, perhaps most highly developed in hospice and palliative care, signals a further expansion of clinical surveillance and medicalization, rather than a liberation from the reductionist tendencies of traditional biomedicine. Armstrong (1983, 1995) has argued, for example, that the recent focus on 'subjectivity' in clinical work is evidence of a paradigmatic shift in the historical development of medicine. Concern with the workings and mechanics of the body has been extended to an interest in facilitating emotional adjustment to, and acceptance and 'awareness' of, the diagnosis of sickness and of dying. Physical problems of disease requiring biomedical attention are now conjoined with 'psycho-social' problems requiring 'therapeutic' monitoring during medical and nursing work. Such therapeutic monitoring encourages the adoption of a particular stance by the patient, and the professional definition of 'normal' and 'abnormal' expressions of suffering. Looking specifically at the operation of the therapeutic gaze in hospice and palliative care, Field's (1996) description of the 'modern role of dying' captures the way in which professional expectations of 'good death' have become a yardstick against which the 'normality' of death and dying may be compared. Similarly, Walter (1994) describes how Kübler-Ross's 'famous five' (1975: 70) stages of grief have become absorbed into the routines of professional therapeutic monitoring and applied in an uncritical manner. This, Walter argues, is to constrain the individual expression of suffering rather than to liberate it. Wendell-Moller (1996) takes a particularly critical stance in connection with the 'normalizing' tendencies of the 'good grief' literature, arguing that these have become a generalized means of containment and control of dying and bereaved people, rather than an individually tailored response to the huge range of human needs associated with death. In these latter writings, medicalization is a feature of all aspects of professional care and therapeutics, albeit subject to subtle transformations according to cultural and historical context.

Reappraising routinization and medicalization

The theses about routinization and medicalization can be read as persuasive and yet depressing. Certainly the relevant commentators seem to have identified a malaise which is also being recognized within the hospice and palliative care movement; the paper by James and Field (1992), for example, has not only been oft-quoted at palliative care conferences, but seems also to have become an examinable subject within the specialty's masters' degrees. Yet an uncritical acceptance of the argument appears to point to the straitjacket of mundane, shallow uniformity: to organizational structures which lose sight of the broad and complex nature of human needs and which ossify in hierarchical systems of power. In one sense, to accept this Weberian argument is to foreclose on further sociological discussion. The routinization of charisma and the bureaucratization which follows present few challenges to interpretation and understanding. Fortunately, the theses are not sufficiently well defended that we can accept them as given. By this we do not mean that the arguments about routinization and medicalization are somehow 'wrong'. And certainly we do not incline to the kind of revisionism which looks for ways to rekindle the conditions which appear to have prevailed 'before' the processes of routinization and medicalization got underway. Rather we are seeking for a more balanced view on these issues.

First, let us consider some of the historical evidence. One of us has already shown in a detailed analysis of the work of Cicely Saunders and her colleagues in the period 1957–67 (Clark 1998a) that some of the problems exposed by the routinization thesis were already anticipated at an early stage. Indeed, even before St Christopher's opened its doors to patients the question of appropriate structures for management which would not destroy innovation and even the matter of succession of leadership were being discussed. Part of the problem with the routinization thesis is that it places too strong an emphasis on *unintended* consequences of action; whereas the historical evidence suggests that there was significant and early engagement with the underlying issues on the part of those involved. In this sense 'routinization' did not creep up from behind, but was rather planned for and anticipated.

Another issue within this was the conscious decision to make religion secondary to medicine within the St Christopher's project. So rather than a fully fledged religious community (which had been considered at one point), St Christopher's took shape as a community of religious *motivation* which could in turn engage with the secular world of health care and service organization. In this sense there has been no moving away from early ideals; rather it has been the case that the early ideals were framed in such a way as to bring about certain results, in particular the wider applicability and expansion of the St Christopher's model in other settings. Important among these was the task of ensuring that the original charismatic vision and leadership was not essential to the organization's continuance.

On these grounds we would question the detail of the 'routinization' thesis and caution against an uncritical reading. Indeed there is an unsatisfactory linearity about the thesis which suggests only one modality of social change in which, if survival is to be ensured, then routinization and bureaucratization must follow. At the same time it is important to identify more precisely the charismatic aspects of key individuals; charisma cannot simply be equated with a 'strong personality'. Bryman (1992) for example proposes a model of charisma in organizations which recognizes some exchange between leaders and followers and in which charisma is socially and deliberately perpetrated to achieve an effect with which charisma is associated. In this sense we see evidence of sociological romanticism in the routinization thesis as it is applied to hospices; perhaps even the belated endorsement of a radicalizing project which is perceived to be running out of steam. In so doing this line of thinking overlooks the significance of routinization as something important to the maintenance of charisma. In other words the two can exist in a mutually reinforcing relationship. Formal organization and charisma, as several contemporary global corporations reveal, are not incompatible phenomena. We should therefore beware the teleology of an artificial separation between the *mission, beliefs* and *values* of hospices and the palliative care movement, on the one hand, and on the other the *activities* and *practices* through which these are constituted.

In 1989 Seale reviewed empirical evidence from evaluative and particip- ant observation studies of the differences between hospital and hospice care in six major areas: medical therapies, psycho-social care, disclosure of prognosis, carer's involvement, in-patient care, and relations between staff. His review reveals the extent of variation both within hospice and palli- ative care services, and hospital care. Further he demonstrates the existence of many similar processes of patient care in hospices and hospitals. A clear example of the latter is the trend towards open disclosure of a terminal prognosis both within hospitals and hospices. As Seale argues, the existence of this similarity suggests that other aspects of care may also be shared. He notes also that observational studies by Field (1989) and Knight and Field (1981) of care given to dying patients in hospital suggest it is possible to deliver 'hospice'-style care within what appear, at first sight, to be highly medicalized environments. Seale draws upon other studies which support this finding, from both the UK and from the USA. An example is research by investigators in Los Angeles (Kane *et al.* 1984) who demonstrated by means of a randomized controlled trial that there was no difference between hospice and hospital care on a broad range of outcome measures, includ- ing patient's anxiety, depression, pain and other cancer-related symptoms, and anxiety and depression in bereaved spouses in post-death follow-up. Further, in this study, the number and type of medical procedures which patients underwent were similar in both settings of care. Seale concludes on the basis of this and other studies that

> The small amount of evidence reviewed here is not adequate to show whether hospice practice in general is different from hospital practice. It leaves open the possibility that there is no difference.
>
> (Seale 1989: 555)

In a later paper however (Seale 1991a), Seale reports on research based on the comparisons of interviews with relatives and others of 45 patients who had received hospice care and 126 who had received conventional care. Some clear differences emerged, leading Seale to conclude:

What the study reveals beyond question is that the process of hospice care, in both in-patient and home care settings, was rather different from conventional care and that hospice care was in many respects seen as valuable . . . it may be concluded from this study that, given the sort of patients who do, in practice, enter hospice care, satisfaction with that care reported by respondents after the death is very high, and generally higher than that of respondents for patients in conventional care.

(Seale 1991a: 151)

Aspects of hospice care that were identified by respondents as particularly valuable were the nursing care received and the less interventionist stance of the medical staff. A small number of other studies has attempted to research differences between hospice and conventional care, concentrating mainly on the impact of hospice-style care on bereavement outcome (Cameron and Murray Parkes 1983; Kane *et al.* 1986; Ransford and Smith 1991), and concluding that particular aspects of hospice style care (facilitation of awareness; adequate pain control; a rehearsal of tasks to be faced after the death; encouragement of family involvement; and bereavement support) had long-term beneficial effects on grief resolution. Such conclusions suggest that, at least at the end of the 1980s, and in certain key respects, hospice care was perceived as qualitatively different from conventional care, and had managed to avoid the reincorporation envisaged by the medicalization and routinization arguments.

More recently, other writers and researchers suggest that the picture may not be quite so clear. Field, writing in 1994, argues that the emergence of palliative medicine as a specialty in 1987 is a manifestation of care given to dying people and evidence of the erosion of hospice style provision. Field expresses five interrelated concerns:

• there is a lack of clarity about the remit of palliative medicine;
• there is a lack of emphasis on dying;
• there is a tendency towards the 'inappropriate' use of technology;
• there is a threat to the autonomy of other health care professionals;
• the role of hospices is threatened by the expansion of palliative medicine.

In a robust response to Field's views, Ahmedzai (1994) argues that lack of clarity of remit and de-emphasis on the terminal stages of illness are strengths rather than weaknesses:

The real issue is not so much: How does palliative medicine differ from terminal care?; but: Which different sections of the population will it open up to humanely applied, scientifically validated care in their hours, days and years of need?

(Ahmedzai 1994: 124)

Ahmedzai is making the point here that there is no simplistic relationship between the use of medical practices and the subversion of hospice principles. It is the purpose behind such practices that is critical; and this extends even to the use of the 'high technology' interventions singled out by Field for special criticism. Ahmedzai suggests that Field's arguments that many hospices are using technology in an inappropriate way is based on an erroneous reading of the results of a survey by Johnson *et al.* (1990), which showed that UK hospices with full-time medical consultants are more likely to use 'high technology' interventions:

> It is by no means clear from a survey like Johnson's that the use of technology is either an appropriate or inappropriate use; one can only say from it that technology is used. It could be on the other hand, in palliative care units where technological interventions are not on offer, that patients are being denied potentially useful tests and therapies.
>
> (Ahmedzai 1994: 124)

The complexities of the relationship between medicine and palliative care principles illustrated by the difference of opinion between Field and Ahmedzai are thrown into sharp relief by the evidence from a recent survey conducted within one hospice of the views of patients and nurses about the value of invasive procedures and tests (Meystre *et al.* 1997). The authors conclude:

> Even patients who are terminally ill are prepared to accept invasive procedures and treatments more readily than their nurses . . . Care must be taken to ensure that the judgements and attitudes of staff are not denying the opportunity of simple tests or therapeutic interventions from which they may benefit.
>
> (Meystre *et al.* 1997: 1202)

These results pose a challenge to the de-medicalization lobby, given the ethics of individual choice, autonomy and empowerment, which underpin the hospice movement. However, the correspondence published in response to Meystre *et al.*'s paper highlights, among other things, the balance that needs to be secured between the ethics of autonomy and the duty of care incumbent upon medical practitioners (Mitchell 1997). Good communication between doctor and patient about the relative values of treatments and tests will ensure that these are used in a judicious and appropriate way, rather than in a futile and inappropriate fashion (Morgan and King 1997; O'Donnell 1997; Stewart *et al.* 1997).

Reviews by Higginson (1993, 1997) and Robbins (1997, 1998) suggest that current changes in the organization of health care make researching the differences between palliative and conventional care subject to a wide range of complex uncertainties and methodological difficulties. Arguments in support of, or against, the emergence of routinization and medicalization become increasingly difficult to establish given the proliferation of palliative care in many different settings of care and the movement of patients with palliative care needs from one care setting to another. As Robbins observes, there has been an '. . . astonishing variation in the pattern and mix of specialist and non specialist, voluntary and statutory services' (1997: 19) in recent years. Such variation may be read by some commentators as evidence of a subversion of hospice principles by the inevitable forces of routinization and medicalization. However, the opposite argument can also be constructed convincingly: that what we are witnessing is the adaptation and growth of a successful social movement which retains its original philosophy and which now is reaping the benefits of its proven ability to influence the mainstream (itself one of the original aims). Seale (1989) examines the former position, acknowledging that the existence of similarities between hospices and hospitals revealed by his review may support the argument that hospices are becoming reincorporated into the bureaucratic machinery and clinical practices of mainstream medical care. However, as Seale argues, this argument serves to conceal the extent to which relationships between people involved in clinical work affect fundamentally the character of the care given to patients and their families. It is to this last point that we now turn.

As Seale points out, observational studies (James 1986; Hockey 1988, 1990; Field 1989) suggest that the quality and nature of interpersonal relationships in various clinical settings are critical influences on the delivery of care to dying and seriously ill people. Clearly such relationships are affected partially by the nature and wider philosophy of the institution in which they are embedded, but the influence is not unidirectional in character. Rather, a dialectical relationship would appear to exist between organizational constraints and goals and the choices, aims and philosophies which direct individual action and which are co-constructed within the interpersonal relationships enacted during clinical work. It is simplistic to suggest that interrelationships within small hospices will be naturally conducive to the delivery of good palliative care. This may indeed be the case, but the opposite may also be true. Field's (1989) work, mentioned above, demonstrates that what may be recognized as effective and sensitive palliative care may be delivered within highly 'conventional' and technical clinical settings such as coronary care units, given appropriate leadership and organization of nursing and medical work. Similarly research in intensive care nursing suggests the existence of many similarities with the philosophy of hospice care nursing, in spite of their apparently opposed circumstances of care delivery (Seymour 1997).

We see little value then in the polarization of debates on routinization and medicalization which are promulgated by revisionist elements within or without the palliative care movement. This should not become a cottage industry for the generation of homespun wisdom. Rather we would encourage further elaboration of the theses through an attention to empirical evidence, which may yet reveal some complex institutional and professional processes at work.

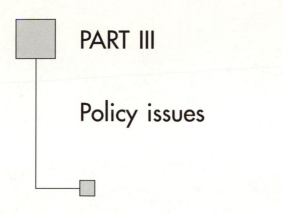

PART III

Policy issues

Introduction to Part III

We have already begun in earlier chapters to touch on matters of policy as they relate to palliative care developments. In Part III we enter into a much fuller discussion of this area. We take a deliberately wide view of what is meant by 'policy' and include within it the processes and activities of government departments, the work of planning and commissioning organizations, and the activities of the agencies which provide health and social care. The early development of hospice and terminal care in Britain seems to have occurred almost in spite of, rather than because of, the interests of policy makers. But over time the hospice and palliative care movement has had to become more interconnected with matters of policy if its goals are to be furthered. In Part III, therefore, the following four areas should be noted particularly:

- The evolving relationship between hospice and palliative care and the National Health Service, with its associated tensions and attempts at partnership.
- The growing impact of wider matters of health and social care policy on the manner in which palliative care is organized and delivered.
- The expansion and diversification of palliative care into a wide variety of settings: hospice; home; hospital; and institutional homes.
- The patchy evidence base for the effectiveness of these services and in particular the lack of research studies which compare directly the benefits of specialist provision with mainstream care.

We begin our exploration of policy issues by showing how the modern hospices relate to the National Health Service. From the outset this was an ambivalent relationship. Much of the focus of the NHS in its early decades was upon the enormous task of coordinating a system of care which was universal in character and free at the point of delivery. The creation of the NHS unlocked a huge flood gate of demand for health care and it quickly became apparent that cost containment would be a matter of central importance to the organization of the service. Acute health care problems and the needs of the chronic sick however were to dominate the agenda.

By the time St Christopher's opened in 1967 the care of the dying had still been largely ignored by the National Health Service as a matter for strategic thinking or planning. The response to St Christopher's and the other independent charitable hospices which followed it was therefore a piecemeal one. The NHS made available grants-in-aid to the early hospices, tolerated their enthusiasms, but did little to harness the burgeoning movement to any strategic purpose. There resulted a rash of uncoordinated developments around the country, which were welcomed within their local communities, but viewed increasingly as a matter of concern by health planners.

As management principles took hold in the NHS, however, through a series of reforms which began in the mid-1970s, so the place of terminal care within the service began to be more clearly defined. Nevertheless, it was not until 1980 that the first official report on the new hospices was produced. The Wilkes Report cautioned against unplanned expansion of independent hospices and argued for greater integration with mainstream services in hospital and the community. But it did little to stem the flow of independent hospice expansion. NHS terminal care services were beginning to appear, but these were again being promoted by cancer charities which provided necessary start-up and revenue funding, for example to support Macmillan continuing care units, as well as Macmillan and Marie Curie Nurses.

By the late 1980s the government was at last requiring district health authorities to take a more strategic view of terminal care. The health authorities were asked to work with the voluntary sector, family practitioner committees and local authorities to ensure that the needs and preferences of terminally ill people were being addressed and that appropriate staff training was available. This was the beginning of what we describe as an *uneasy alliance* between the hospice and palliative care movement and the NHS. Soon special ring-fenced monies were available for the voluntary hospices; but their allocation was controversial and appeared to discriminate against NHS services. Ring-fencing of funds was incompatible however with the increasing market orientation of the health service. In the early 1990s palliative care was faced with the task of adapting to fundamental changes in the NHS which brought about an internal market for care in which the functions of purchasers and providers were radically separated.

The conservative reforms of the NHS of the early 1990s brought many implications for the hospices and for palliative care more generally. An era of contracts, audit and quality assurance was ushered in, to which palliative care showed considerable alacrity in adapting. There was also a growing emphasis on user involvement, on needs assessment and upon equity of access. In particular interest grew in the extension of palliative care to people with non-malignant conditions, with 'palliative care for all' as the rallying call. We discuss all of these points in detail here, together with other matters of health policy which impacted upon palliative care in these years, such as general practitioner fundholding; the new arrangements for continuing care; and the Calman-Hine rationalizations of cancer services.

It was in this unfolding policy arena that palliative care services were expanding and diversifying from the early 1970s onwards. In Part III we therefore review this broad programme of service development, focusing on the different settings in which care is delivered.

Hospital-based provision of palliative care has been a major challenge for the specialty, but numerous studies have pointed to the need for improving care in this setting. The first hospital-based palliative care teams began in Britain in the late 1970s. They have taken various forms and differ considerably in the extent to which they have multidisciplinary involvement. Undoubtedly, such teams have the ability to offer good coverage of need – they are located in the same place as some of the most ill people in the health care system. Yet a picture continues to emerge of their work being pursued against the odds and without systematic support from health authorities and trusts. One difficulty which they must overcome is that of providing substantial evidence of their efficacy; and the paucity of systematic research on their activities is surprisingly marked.

Palliative care at home is the stated policy aim of many health care commissioners and providers. Here we see the paradox that most people wish to die at home, but only a minority achieve their preference. Recent evidence has brought attention to the particular problems of those dying at home with non-malignant conditions. The primary health care teams are of course at the centre of health care in the community and we discuss how they relate to other generic services, particularly in the context of the needs of informal carers.

One feature of the expansion of palliative care has been the rise of specialist domiciliary services. At times these have found it difficult to establish close working relationships with the primary health care teams, but studies of palliative care at home have produced encouraging results. For some patients who are living at home with advanced disease, access to hospice day care is an importance service. We trace the development of hospice day care services, and note their popularity with independent providers, but again draw attention to the lack of research evidence on their efficacy, and their particular service claims in a context where day care provision by a wide variety of non-palliative care agencies is now in evidence.

We then turn to the particular service setting where modern palliative care originated – the in-patient hospice. Over 200 hospice units now exist in the United Kingdom and the numbers continue to expand, albeit more modestly than in earlier years. In recent times there has been a pattern of growing integration between hospices and other local health care providers. We discuss the coverage which the hospices achieve of those in need within their local populations and the types of care which they offer. The future of hospices is a topic to which we return in our conclusion. We conclude Part III however with a discussion of care at the end of life in institutional homes of various kinds. There was a huge proliferation of these in the course of the 1990s and some 15 per cent of all deaths now occur there. Some such homes aspire to the provision of high-quality palliative care, but in general, standards of care in such settings remain an object of concern.

So in Part III we have attempted a wide-ranging review of questions of strategic planning and service delivery as they relate to hospice care, terminal care and palliative care in the United Kingdom since the beginning of the National Health Service. We draw attention to the following themes as matters of key importance: the unfolding relationship between the NHS and the palliative care movement; the increasing interrelations between palliative care and matters of mainstream health and social policy; the rapid expansion and diversification of palliative care services; and the lack of evidence about the 'added value' of palliative care.

7 Policy development and palliative care

As we saw in Chapter 4 it was the British post-war policy context which formed the backdrop to the first growth points of the modern hospice movement. Subsequently British health policy has undergone some important transitions as successive governments have sought simultaneously to demonstrate to the electorate their support for the National Health Service whilst also trying to bring the service within manageable limits of organization and cost. The early hospice leaders were disinclined to be fettered by matters of policy; after all here was a social movement which was seeking to counterpose itself to some aspects of the dominant system. At the same time they could never fully escape the constraints of policy and coexistence with the prevailing arrangements soon became a matter for acceptance. Subsequently we can trace a growing interconnectedness between hospice care, palliative care and health and social care more generally. We discussed some of the implications of this for models of care in Chapters 5 and 6. In recent years this trend has continued to such an extent that it is now quite impossible to form a view on the current state of palliative care without also turning to matters of policy.

At this point it is worth expanding a little on what we mean by 'policy'. Levin (1997) draws attention to the slipperiness of the concept. Politicians and academics frequently disagree on what they mean by 'policy'. As Levin points out, politicians make several claims about policy: as a stated intention; a current or past action; an organizational practice; or as an indicator of the formal status of a particular course of action (1997: 15). For politicians, policy also has certain attributes, denoting belongingness; commitment; status; and specificity (1997: 17). Politicians also *enact* policy, through legislative measures, decisions about public expenditure, organizational structuring and management activities. Academics however are inclined to more abstract definitions of policy. For them policy may be a course of action, or of inaction, or it may be a statement about the goals of society and the means of achieving them. As Levin points out these academic definitions may fail to capture those features of policy which are most salient to politicians (1997: 24). Both views are helpful however.

In our experience much of the debate about how policy impacts upon palliative care has focused on the nature of commitments made by government, the extent to which they will be honoured and the mechanisms for their enactment. The case of 50–50 funding for hospices, shared between government and the voluntary sector (to which we return later in this chapter), is a classic example. Palliative care conferences involving key providers and professional groups are often places where such issues are debated. Indeed it may be one marker of the 'routinization' of hospice care that its practitioners have become absorbed increasingly with such matters of policy. Less commonly heard are the bigger questions: where does palliative care fit into a range of goals concerning the well-being and quality of life of all citizens within a society and how can it best be organized in relation to such goals? Indeed we might say again that the absence of such questions – which certainly did concern the early hospice founders – may also be taken as a marker of the assimilation of palliative care into the mainstream of health care delivery.

For these reasons we want to offer here an approach to policy which is wide-ranging in character, which encompasses the views of multiple stakeholders and which also retains a concern with values. Margaret Stacey has captured exactly these concerns in her discussion of health policy and the sociological contribution to understanding it:

> By health policy I understand those managerial, collective or aggregated individual decisions which affect the way in which health care is delivered. Health policy thus includes the care and treatment policies developed by consultant clinicians, nurses, midwives and their teams, firms or divisions. It also includes the policies promulgated by general managers, health authorities, the Department of Health and those in charge of private health-care arrangements. It is important, I think, to recognise that policy decisions are taken at all levels from those of government, which have the most global effect, to those which directly impact on the treatment patients in a particular facility may receive. Mine may be a broader definition than that taken by some policy analysts, but it is of the nature of the division of health labour that health-care policy emerges from all these decision-making locales. Furthermore, sociology can be and is applied to policies at all these levels. If this is not recognised, an inadequate account of the sociological contribution results.
>
> (Stacey 1991: 14)

In this chapter and those which follow therefore we shall focus on multiple understandings of 'policy' as it relates to palliative care. By doing this we hope to capture a sense of what palliative care means to different groups of people: those who provide it; those who make use of it; those responsible for funding and organizing it; and, ultimately that wider group of citizens, the general population, whose overall well-being it is intended to serve. In this chapter we examine how palliative care is planned nationally and procured locally and what information is used to inform the configuration of available services.

The NHS and the early hospices

The questions of for whom, by whom and in what ways health care should be delivered have been central to the UK National Health Service since its inception and are also entirely familiar to other health care systems around the world. The National Health Service at the time of its establishment in 1948 however was unique. Offering free medical care to the entire population, it was a comprehensive system of universal entitlement. It represented collective provision for health care within a market economy (Klein 1983). Underpinning it was the replacement of charity, dependency and moralism as well as the bureaucratic surveillance of private lives, with a new ethic of social citizenship (Harris 1996). Its organization from the outset however was a matter of immense complexity.

Webster's monumental history of the NHS points out that

> Given the precipitous and haphazard manner in which the NHS was put together, there was no opportunity to incorporate arrangements for comprehensive and integrated planning, or even to guarantee the efficient use of resources.
>
> (Webster 1996: 27)

Many of the flawed principles of financial management of pre-NHS bodies were simply imported uncritically into the new service. At the same time the Ministry of Health was from the outset under pressure to contain costs, so that by 1958 Titmuss could state: 'Any general impression that the Health Service is entirely a "free" service . . . requires correction' (Titmuss 1958: 138). Dental, ophthalmic and prescription charges were soon established and by the tenth anniversary of the NHS there was widespread discussion about other potential charges: for ambulance services; 'hotel' costs in hospital; and restrictions on available drugs (Timmins 1996: 204). Tensions in the system, however, were not only financial.

The NHS had grown out of a slowly emerging consensus. One aspect of this was reflected in its organizational structures. There was a nervousness about excessive centralization and a devolved approach to administration had been adopted in order to reassure interest groups anxious about excessive control from Whitehall. During the 1950s there were thus some '800 autonomous units of health service administration' all 'in danger of replicating the omissions, duplications and inefficiencies which characterised the prewar health services, and which the NHS was designed to correct' (Webster 1996: 29). The problem was seen to rest within the 'tripartite system' of hospital services, executive council services and local authority services. Nonetheless, the system remained substantially unchanged for the first quarter century of the NHS's existence.

It was into this system that the first of the modern hospices in Britain emerged. Like the NHS itself, the hospices contained conflicting tendencies. On the one hand they were progressive and modernizing, seeking to improve care of the dying through new methods of pain and symptom management. On the other hand they harked back to the very world of charity and voluntarism which the NHS had sought to supersede. The early hospices from St Christopher's onwards were independent charities: they raised funds for capital development and subsidized their costs through charitable giving and voluntary labour. At the same time they also looked to hospital boards for the funding of beds. As Cicely Saunders puts it in an article marking the opening of the first modern hospice: 'St Christopher's Hospice is outside the National Health Service; but it has contractual arrangements with a regional hospital board and a grant from the Ministry for research into pain' (1967: 988). Wilkes, writing in 1981, captures the spirit of setting up a hospice in Sheffield some 15 years earlier:

> The regional hospital board agreed that such a unit was needed but said that they could not possibly afford to build it. They did agree, however, that if we raised the money to build from private sources they would help generously with the running costs. Of course they would not promise this now. Even then, I suspect, they agreed because they thought we would never raise the money...
>
> (Wilkes 1981: 1591)

In this way the enthusiasm of charismatic pioneers, like Wilkes and Saunders, both doctors and both emerging as experts in the new field of terminal care, were to win the day with less informed, bureaucratically cautious administrators in the health service. Part of the difficulty for the administrators, of course, was that of being seen to be opposing something so emotive as the care of the dying. Indeed the early pioneers constructed a self-conscious moral case for their cause in their various writings. Thus Cicely Saunders could note as early as 1961 that 'A society which shuns the dying must have an incomplete philosophy' (Saunders 1961: np). Or likewise, Wilkes, in a remark on research but which could just as easily have been aimed at the planners, noted: 'You cannot calibrate suffering' (Wilkes 1965: 799). By such means an era of *emotional planning* gathered momentum. Within this a growing number of local hospice initiatives, many inspired by the writings and teachings of Cicely Saunders and often linked to individual experiences of poor terminal care, got underway. Such initiatives quickly captured the public imagination. Health service planners were taken unawares. Agreements to support the hospices were made on an *ad hoc* basis with no clear conception of where such developments might lead. The rapid expansion of hospices, mainly in the independent sector, already described in Chapter 4, therefore took place in spite, rather than because, of NHS planning. At this stage the NHS had been indifferent to the care of the dying, caught up with many other pressures and demands. Paradoxically, the vacuum of indifference was filled by an emergent voluntary hospice movement, which over time would become a source of concern to the planners whose very quietude had fuelled its expansion.

Charitable giving and the establishment of new independent hospices were closely interconnected. Local groups could raise funds for the 'bricks and mortar' of a hospice which would be established as a visible sign of care within the community. Popular commentary has described this as 'amongst the highest levels of giving in a community' (Lewis 1989: 67). Likewise it could be seen as 'highly motivated and caring people from many walks of life, bringing valuable experience to bear on a very specialised problem on which expert guidance has not always been readily available' (Harper *et al.* 1989: 2). Only gradually did such guidance begin to appear.

By 1979 hospice services were growing rapidly, but in an unplanned manner. Looking back to that year, Lunt observed:

> There were many voluntary groups around the country who, inspired by the success of St Christopher's Hospice, were collecting money 'to build a hospice', often with very little idea precisely how this was going to meet the needs of their particular community, how it would fit in with other kinds of provision locally and elsewhere . . . The DHSS had no policy. There was no monitoring of the growth of these services. Attempts to plan or co-ordinate services were made difficult by the lack of any systematic information on what services existed, on what scale and with what to offer. Information was also lacking on the scale of provision which might be required to meet the needs of any given population.
>
> (Lunt 1985: 754)

In the following years the 'visionary' and the 'bureaucratic' (Clark 1993b) systems of hospice founders and NHS planners, respectively, were to co-exist in a state of tension. For the planners, expanding hospice numbers required an uneasy accommodation to the continuing role of charitable ideals within the NHS. For hospice visionaries there was the growing realization that coexistence with the NHS and some degree of collaboration with it would be a key to longer term survival.

Managing the NHS and managing terminal care

The NHS too had been changing in these years. Under the original system of 1948 the hospital boards ran the hospitals (and so it was these to which the early hospices looked for support). It was the local authorities however which were responsible for district nursing, health visiting, midwifery, maternity, child welfare and other community services. Under successive governments there had been discussions of various alternative options. In 1974 700 hospital boards, boards of governors, management committees and executive councils disappeared. They were replaced by 14 regional health authorities, 90 area health authorities, each linked with a family practitioner committee, and 200 district management teams, each with a community health council to watch over it. It was an 'organisational monstrosity' described by Timmins as 'imbued with the latest outputs of fashionable management theory' (1996: 295). There was to be 'maximum delegation downwards', coupled with 'maximum accountability upwards', all held together by principles of 'consensus management'. As Strong and Robinson put it:

> The new management tiers had, in turn, a new management ethos. An elaborate planning system was created, based on current management fashion. The administrative rhythm in each region, area and district soon came to centre round the endless construction and varying cycles of detailed plans.
>
> (Strong and Robinson 1990: 17)

However, for the first time there were health authorities responsible for planning health services for their populations. The changes had been engineered by a Conservative government, with Sir Keith Joseph as the Minister. They came into force however under a brief period of government by Labour, which decided to let them stand. The following years also saw some attempts to equalize health care spending in order to erode the high funding differential which existed between districts and regions in different parts of the country. This RAWP (Resource Allocation Working Party) mechanism was also linked to other redistributive measures – in particular the move to shift resources from the acute sector into community and long-term care (Strong and Robinson 1990: 12–13).

The burgeoning hospices were therefore having to liaise with a National Health Service which was becoming more managerialist, more strategic and better coordinated. Gaining support from the hospital board in order to promote the cause of a local hospice was now replaced by liaison with the area or district health authority. At area level a new vantage point was available from which to view the array of local services and plan for the future. Hospices thus became part of a bigger picture, even at local level, where the services they offered could be seen alongside others in both the in-patient and community settings.

A landmark of policy recognition for the hospices came in 1980 with the publication of the report of the Working Group on Terminal Care (1980), produced by the Standing Subcommittee on Cancer of the Standing Medical Advisory Committee. Generally known as 'the Wilkes Report', after its chairperson, this was a document prepared against a background of proliferation in the numbers of in-patient hospices. It was evidence of the significant developments which had taken place in the 20 years since Glyn Hughes (1960) had called for more homes for the dying. Wilkes and his colleagues were of the opinion, however, that limits to the growth of specialized hospices would be imposed both by the lack of suitable staff to work in them and by a scarcity of the necessary revenue funding. They also were unsure about the wisdom of 'hiding away' dying people in special homes detached from wider services. In a bold statement the working group therefore took the view that it did 'not consider that there would be any advantage in promoting a large increase in the number of hospices at present', preferring instead to 'encourage the dissemination of the principles of terminal care throughout the health service and to develop an integrated system of care with emphasis on coordination between the primary care sector, the hospital sector and the hospice movement' (Working Group on Terminal Care 1980: 10). Under these arrangements increased attention would be given to home care and to day care. In the event the working group was proved both right and wrong. Certainly, there followed a huge dissemination of what was to become palliative care into other sectors of the health service; but the number of specialist in-patient units also trebled in the decade after the report's publication.

Undertaken in the same year that the Wilkes Report was published, a survey by Lunt and Hillier (1981) showed that 58 in-patient units were now in existence, but also that 32 home care teams had been created, together with eight hospital support teams. Regional differences in provision continued to be significant and the authors made recommendations: that home care teams should take priority over in-patient units; that hospital support teams should be encouraged; and that future services within each region should be coordinated to ensure the most beneficial combination of voluntary and NHS provision.

At this point a large national charity, the National Society for Cancer Relief (NSCR, now Macmillan) began its own efforts to stimulate and coordinate development. A repeat of the earlier survey showed that between December 1980 and August 1983, 55 new services had been established, mainly in home and hospital settings. Over three-quarters of these services (78 per cent) had been funded by the NSCR and the majority were located in the poorly provided regions. Less encouragingly however, NHS mainstream funding of terminal care remained almost static in these years (Lunt 1985).

In 1987 the government published its first official circular on terminal care (Department of Health 1987). Along with subsequent guidance which appeared in the ensuing years, it made a number of points clear. District health authorities would take the lead in planning and coordinating a comprehensive and integrated range of services for terminally ill people. Districts would also ensure, in consultation with the voluntary sector, family practitioner committees and local authorities, that mechanisms were in place to assess the needs and preferences of clients, and to identify deficiencies in services and staff training. Clear strategies, with monitoring arrangements, should be produced in all districts. A key focus of this guidance was the problem of identifying a long-term funding mechanism for the voluntary hospices. Indeed, by 1989 public concerns were being expressed that the hospices would not be able to meet the increased salary costs resulting from nurse regradings then taking place across the NHS, unless some £4.5 million was forthcoming from government. By now Help the Hospices had been established for five years as an umbrella charity to support hospice developments; it also began to lobby government.

An uneasy alliance

The next step in the unfolding policy response to the hospices had substantial and controversial effects. Following a ministerial statement in late 1989, it became apparent that the government's intention was for 'health authorities to work towards a full partnership which matches the voluntary giving towards hospice services' (Department of Health 1990: 1). New monies of £8 million accompanied this statement, bringing government support for hospice revenues to an estimated £20 million (Department of Health 1990: 1). By 1993 the figure had more than doubled to £43 million. Nevertheless, there were problems. First the government had entered into a commitment to a 50–50 funding model which could have the effect of fuelling rather than curtailing the unplanned developments which had become an object of concern. Second, the commitment appeared open-ended: would government continue to match pound for pound the contributions from charitable sources, with no ceiling? Third, and crucially, the scheme was divisive; these new monies, announced year on year in the early 1990s were 'ring-fenced' to the voluntary sector only. They appeared to discriminate against palliative care services planned and delivered within the NHS. Not surprisingly, the scheme led to much debate (Clark 1991, 1993c). It seemed to provoke an unseemly scramble for resources among independent hospices. NHS services looked for legitimate ways to access the funds in partnership with charitable bodies which could make application on their behalf. As one of us noted at the time, the allocations, via the regional health authorities, 'caused a good deal of controversy within the hospice world: local competition for available funds, lack of clarity about criteria for eligibility, allegations of underspending by regions' (Clark 1993c:

170). Above all, the scheme was at odds with the new market orientation to health care which was becoming so central to government policy. Ministers found it difficult to defend in public (Clark 1993b: 9) and it proved complex to administer. Although much liked by the independent hospices themselves, who sought to preserve it, the scheme was first widened to include NHS palliative care services before eventually being dropped in 1995. Henceforth, monies for hospice and palliative care services were to be found from within health authorities' baseline budgets. Ring-fencing of funds, with its associations of protectionism, was over. During the five years in which the scheme operated the government shifted its rationale from '50–50 partnership' to 'preparation for contracts'. There were now bigger changes taking place in the NHS than ever before and these would soon have a direct bearing on the world of hospice and palliative care.

With the landslide Conservative victory of 1979 and Margaret Thatcher as Prime Minister, a new set of questions about the NHS came onto the agenda. In the following years the welfare state was to come 'under fire' (Timmins 1996: 369). A policy debate began to emerge which emphasized reforming the supply side of the economy, reducing marginal tax rates, reshaping the labour market and controlling the welfare budget (Pierson 1996: 154). The NHS, of course, was a highly sensitive political target, even for an ideologically driven government of the New Right cushioned by a large parliamentary majority. Butler (1994) sees three issues at play here. First was the paramount importance of a sound economy: social policy would always be subservient to economic well-being. Second, there was the conviction that nothing should be done by the public sector that might be done just as well in the private sector. Third was an 'axiomatic assumption' (Butler 1994: 14) of organizational inefficiency born out of vested interests and protectionism. Key NHS changes of the 1980s therefore have to be understood in the light of these broader policy convictions. It was the 1980s which finally saw the introduction of general management into the NHS in a bid to displace public sector bureaucratic inefficiency with private sector values and practices. This move would prove particularly important to the development of the internal market following the health reforms of the next decade. Other changes in the 1980s however included the introduction of schemes for income generation and the principle of contracting out for key ancillary services.

The principles of general management within the NHS were first enunciated in a report written by Sir Roy Griffiths, the head of the supermarket chain Sainsbury's. His report highlighted the obscurity of management within the service and contained a phrase that was to be much quoted subsequently: 'If Florence Nightingale were carrying her lamp through the corridors of the NHS today she would almost certainly be searching for the people in charge' (DHSS 1983: 12). Griffiths set out to complete the unfinished business of the 1974 reforms to the NHS. In each tier of management (region, district, unit) a single leader, or general manager, was installed. The NHS itself was also given a management board, with a chief executive, and each region now had a general manager. As Strong and Robinson put it: 'There was, for the first time, a single line of command from the top to the bottom of the service' (1990: 23). As a result: 'the clinical trades fell, the others rose' (1990: 25). Where administration had once existed, now 'management' prevailed. Consensus had lost out to control in a service which was soon set for even more sweeping alterations.

Most commentators agree that the reforms embodied in the 1990 NHS and Community Care Act constitute 'the greatest change in the organisation and management of the NHS since it was established' (Robinson 1994: 2). For the first time the functions of purchasing and providing health care services were separated out. On the demand side District Health Authorities *and* general practice fundholders held budgets to procure appropriate services on behalf of their populations. On the supply side the key players became newly formed NHS trusts; but much greater recognition was given than ever before to the role of not-for-profit and private health care providers. There was to be a mixed economy of care aimed to reduce reliance on state provision. Primary care was again given more prominence as were the principles and practice of community care. Market thinking and analogies became a part of NHS systems and the principles of general management with associated business ethics and ideas were given even fuller extent. The values underpinning this were rooted strongly in new right ideologies. State care was costly, inefficient and poorly planned; it must be subjected to the rigours of market forces. Likewise health and illness were reconstructed as matters of personal responsibility and lifestyle, 'consumers' of health care should therefore be encouraged to take change of their own needs and also to be more discriminating in their use of services. With this in mind there would be a much greater emphasis upon clinical audit, quality assurance, complaints procedures and the views of local people.

The Conservative reforms and palliative care

In a number of earlier papers produced in Sheffield, we have argued that the key to understanding the Conservative reforms to the NHS in the 1990s lies in the purchasing cycle (Neale *et al.* 1994; Clark *et al.* 1995; Clark *et al.* 1997b). Existing as a model for the organization of an internal 'quasi market' (Flynn *et al.* 1995) the purchasing cycle provides us with a view of two essential policy elements: *efficiency* of operation and *effectiveness* of impact. It comprises five key components (Clark *et al.* 1997b): health needs assessment; purchasing strategy; service specification; contracting; and quality assurance. By such means health services in a local district are predicated upon a clear analysis of the need for them; they form part of an overall strategic vision; within this specific elements of required services can be detailed; a contractual agreement is then reached with a named provider of the service in question; and the provision of services is subsequently monitored for quality and quantity within an agreed framework. This was the essential framework set in place by the NHS reforms of the early 1990s, and it was to this set of policy arrangements that palliative care would, increasingly, have to respond.

In 1992 another expert committee on palliative care had reported its findings (SMAC/SNMAC 1992). Interestingly, and unlike the Wilkes Report, this was not produced by a standing medical committee on cancer, but by a combined committee of doctors and nurses, reporting to the Minister. Although lacking the radicalism of its predecessor, the new report did seek to deal with the overall 'positioning' of hospice services in relation to a widening array of palliative care provision. A key feature of this report was the recommendation that greater effort should be made to extend palliative care services to diagnostic groups beyond cancer and that palliative care should be provided on an individualized basis, wherever it is required, rather than solely in specialized units. The report did seek to clarify a number of key terms in the ever more differentiated lexicon of palliative care. It also made a total of 20 recommendations covering general principles: strategy, organization and provision together with education, research and audit. Two main foundations for success were identified. First, education for health professionals in palliative care should be available at all levels. Second, the new purchasing authorities must define population needs and develop appropriate services in relation to them, delivered as an integrated whole within the NHS. The voluntary hospices were scarcely mentioned. Nevertheless, the report would be used subsequently by both purchasers and providers to define an agenda for how palliative care services should be developing at district level. These discussions were strengthened in turn by the growing volume of academic and professional commentary on palliative care. Journals, conferences and professional bodies proliferated. In 1987 palliative medicine had been recognized as a specialty and in 1991 the National Council for Hospice and Specialist Palliative Care Services was formed. Both helped to ensure that palliative care developments in the 1990s would be accompanied by closer scrutiny and more sophisticated commentary than had the events of the previous decade.

For most palliative care commentators and policy analysts, purchasing issues were a major object of interest in the middle years of the 1990s. A number of issues caused concern. There was the question of how general practice fundholding, and later the 'total purchasing' pilot schemes, would affect palliative care providers. Much discussion centred around the arbitrary divisions which the new legislation had created between 'health' and 'social' care, and the associated 'shunting' of costs between them, particularly in relation to continuing care needs. There was also anxiety about the impact of ring-fence removal from the special monies government had been setting aside for palliative care. In due course the impact of the Calman-Hine Report on cancer services (Expert Advisory Group on Cancer 1995) also began to work through into palliative care, most noticeably as the government changed in 1997 and a new White Paper appeared on the NHS. We shall turn to these points in due course, but first let us consider how hospices and specialist palliative care responded more generally to the Conservative NHS reforms of the 1990s, and to the purchasing cycle in particular.

A review of the impact of the reforms on palliative care by 1995 concluded that substantial progress had been made in some areas, a good deal less in others and that the glass might be 'half full' or 'half empty' depending upon the observer's value position and willingness to make a judgement (Clark et al. 1997b). Most positively, there was substantial evidence that palliative care services, many of them delivered by independent voluntary hospices, had quickly established a place within the contract culture. Whereas in the early 1990s hospices had questioned the viability and wisdom of entering into contracts with purchasers, by 1995 these were a universal norm, with an estimated 97 per cent of palliative care services receiving some income from NHS contracts. Less optimistically however, almost one third (31 per cent) of providers had a poor or very poor opinion of their contract. On the question of district health authorities' strategies for palliative care, progress was less marked. Bearing in mind that the formulation of strategic plans of this kind had been a district requirement since 1987, eight years later it was estimated that just over a half (56 per cent) had produced such plans. Worryingly, one palliative care provider in five (21 per cent) had no involvement in the local strategic plan. Finally, on needs assessment, again something pre-figured in the 1987 palliative care circular and given much more prominence in the general policy guidance issued along with the 1989 White Paper, the position was evenly balanced. By 1995 almost exactly one half of purchasers (49 per cent) had conducted a needs assessment specifically for palliative care (Clark et al. 1997b). There was evidence from this study then of considerable enthusiasm for the reforms on the part of specialist palliative care providers, but as with earlier aspects of hospice history, some doubts about the extent to which this was being matched by those within the NHS with responsibility for commissioning palliative care.

Even those critical of the overall orientation and purpose of the Conservative reforms of the NHS have found in the area of needs assessment something about which to be more positive. The idea that health care services should be predicated upon a rational assessment of need rather than upon emotional pleading, political lobbying, or the vested interests of particular providers is one with which it is difficult to disagree. Of course, such rational assessment presents many challenges and some of these are particularly marked in the case of palliative care.

Stevens and Raftery acknowledge that needs assessment 'means different things according to who uses the term, when and where' (1997: xi). There is a welcome pluralism about this, for needs assessment will always contain political and value positions and cannot be viewed from a purely positivist perspective. How questions about need are constructed, the instruments which are used to measure it and the actions which flow can never be purely detached matters of disinterested science. Rather they are likely to be contested territory open to a variety of viewpoints. This should not detract from the value of a rational approach, but such rationalism should be tempered by an awareness of the social dimensions influencing the 'science' of needs assessment.

First we must acknowledge that there are certain conceptual difficulties surrounding the definition of need and its value for policy purposes. Stevens and Raftery define health care need as 'the population's ability to bene-fit from health care' (1997: xi). From here they are able to identify two essential components of a population's ability to benefit: first, the incidence and prevalence of a health problem; second, the effectiveness of the inter-ventions available to deal with it. This also involves distinguishing need from demand ('what people would be willing to pay for or might wish to use in a system of free health care') and from supply ('what is actually provided') (Stevens and Raftery 1997: xii). In general, we know a great deal more about demand and supply than we do about need.

As needs assessment entered into the lexicon of health service planning in the 1990s, a number of palliative care analysts and commentators turned their attention to the subject. An early paper came from the National Council for Hospice and Specialist Palliative Care Services (NCHSPCS 1993). Here we see highlighted the tension between an approach which looks at population need, versus one focused on individuals. Clearly the former was the responsibility of the newly constituted health care purchasers, but for practitioners the centre of attention will be the needs of the indi-vidual. Palliative care of course seeks to look beyond physical needs, so the question of emotional and social needs is also introduced. Likewise the focus of care may go beyond the patient, to include the needs of informal carers. In such a way the assessment of palliative care needs starts to become a rather complex matrix.

Some of this discussion drew on Bradshaw's (1972) earlier distinction between 'felt need' (subjective feelings of individuals), 'normative need' (expert consensus on the matter)' and 'comparative need' (the differing needs of groups of people in similar circumstances). At the same time a more recent paper by Bradshaw had argued that 'the concept of need has always been too imprecise, too complex, too contentious to be a useful target for policy' (1996: 45). Others however were more optimistic about the potential for needs assessment, seeing it as both a political process and a technical activity which could guide decision making and resource allocation (Øvretveit 1995). As Clark and Malson pointed out, however, in the policy context needs were 'increasingly couched in the language of priorities, addressing questions such as who is to have first claim on limited resources and who is to judge that claim?' (1995: 54). The same authors also cautioned against a purely functional concept of need (i.e. that needs only exist where there is a service available to meet them). This they argued was 'a dangerous teleology which is calculated to overlook needs that are difficult to conceptualise, identify or respond to' (1995: 54). In palliative care, for example, needs relating to psychological or spiritual suffering might come into this category, but so too might the needs of underprivileged groups, the socially marginalized or the quiescent. One view might be that the hospice and palliative care movement's particular strength has been to give voice to a previously ignored or misunderstood need. As we have already seen in this chapter that voice was first articulated outside the mainstream of NHS services. Bearing in mind such a history it is reasonable to ask whether the task of assessing need (which as we now see is also about defining need) can safely be left in the hands of those who are responsible for either purchasing or providing current services. In this sense the views of the wider public come into play.

Some approaches to needs assessment acknowledge this and take into account a broad range of perspectives. Clark and Malson saw three components within their model of health needs assessment for palliative care. First is the familiar territory of public health and planning: epidemiological and demographic data. Second, there are comparative data relating to the costs, outputs and outcomes of services. Linking these is a third strand, of *stakeholder perspectives*. Key stakeholders in local palliative care services might include service users (patients and informal carers); providers (of both health and social care); those charged with responsibilities for the funding, organization and planning of services; and also local community groups (with or without a specialist interest in health). This dimension of stakeholder perspectives is of course a potentially challenging one, for the views of different groups may not be in harmony. What it does provide however is a more wide-ranging analysis of how palliative care needs are perceived in a particular locality.

Some studies in the 1990s went on to adopt this kind of multi-layered approach to palliative care needs assessment within specific districts. An early example in Nottingham for instance (Nicholas and Frankenberg 1992) involved surveys of patients and relatives and community and support groups of various kinds as well as an analysis of the views of GPs, consultants, nurses and social workers in the district. A similar project was carried out in the adjacent locality of Southern Derbyshire (Clark *et al.* 1996). Here interviews with members of various community groups revealed several concerns: breaking bad news was perceived to be 'a lottery' in which the chances of being told by a skilled and sensitive practitioner was not guaranteed; there was a lack of information about special conditions and the availability of self-help groups; bereavement care was considered in need of improvement; there were concerns about a lack of choice about the care on offer; and ethnic minority needs and information requirements relating to palliative care were highlighted particularly. The latter issue became a matter of broader concern during the mid-1990s and the growing interest in needs assessment allowed it to be explored further.

A report published by the National Council for Hospice and Specialist Palliative Care Services (NCHSPCS 1995b) focused on the question of how access to hospice and palliative care services could be improved for members of the black and ethnic minority communities. Several factors were seen to contribute to a perceived low take-up of specialist palliative care services on the part of ethnic minority groups: a lack of accurate data on the ethnicity of service users; the younger age profile of ethnic minority populations; a lower incidence of cancer than within the wider population; and a lack of relevant information for potential service users in the ethnic minorities. The report went on to recommend better ethnic monitoring; equal opportunities and antidiscriminatory policies, linked to staff training; and a more culturally specific approach to service provision (NCHSPCS 1995b).

By such means it was possible to begin to incorporate the views of a wider range of stakeholders into the thinking about palliative care needs assessment. Inevitably perhaps the epidemiologically based paradigm remained dominant, albeit broadened to include rather more than socio-demographic and disease-specific data. By 1997, and drawing on a wide range of related studies, it was possible for Higginson to produce an overview of the needs assessment field relating to palliative and terminal care (Higginson 1997). A key point was made on the scale of the problem:

> Within a population of 1,000,000 there are approximately 2,800 cancer deaths per year and of these 2,400 people will experience pain, 1,300 will have trouble with breathing and 1,400 will have symptoms of vomiting or nausea in the last year of life. There will be approximately 6,900 deaths due to progressive non malignant disease and some of these will have had a period of advancing progressive disease when palliative care would have been appropriate. Four thousand, six hundred people will have suffered pain, 3,400 will have had trouble with breathing and 1,900 will have had symptoms of vomiting or nausea in the last year of life.
>
> (Higginson 1997: 1)

Of course a great deal is missing from this assessment of need: psychosocial problems, the experience of informal carers and the wide range of practical and material difficulties which may arise at the end of life.

Nevertheless, it provides a picture of the broad parameters within a health district of typical size. In such districts the assessment of palliative care needs constitutes just one area of concern for those responsible for procuring services. Many of the palliative care policy debates of the 1990s demonstrate how other issues impact on the problem at hand and how palliative care cannot be seen in isolation from other pressing matters in the delivery of health and social care.

Some key issues in the 1990s

We have acknowledged at several points in this chapter that across its history one orientation of policy within the NHS has been a move towards more primary care. The Conservative reforms of the 1990s pressed this further when, in introducing the system of purchasers and providers, the government also brought forward the idea of the fundholding general practice. This would give to general practitioners the capacity to buy hospital services on behalf of their patients. It was another example of a market solution to a health care problem (Glennerster *et al.* 1994: 7). In a scheme introduced in 1991 practices with more than 9000 patients could apply for fundholding status and would receive a budget allocation to be spent on a defined set of purposes. Later the practice size was reduced and the scope of fundholding was extended. General practitioners could thus purchase hospital in-patient care for certain operations; all outpatient visits, including for diagnostic tests; pharmaceuticals prescribed by the practice; community health services, including district nursing, health visiting, chiropody, dietetics; mental health services and services for people with disabilities. Palliative and terminal care were excluded (Glennerster *et al.* 1994). By 1994 the model was extended to a set of pilot practices which would be endowed with total fundholding powers, to cover all services, including palliative care (Department of Health 1994).

Such fundholders were of course viewed with interest by palliative care providers. It emerged that not all of those within the pilot schemes would be intending to purchase palliative care services and one observer noted that the typical general practitioner might see only two patients in a year with specialist palliative care needs (NCHSPCS 1994). This article summarized concerns about general practice fundholding, including the administrative costs of contracting with several fundholders; the resultant difficulties in planning ahead; the percentage of voluntary hospice in-patient bed costs payable to general practitioners in relation to the government's '50–50' commitment; problems in coordinating needs assessment between fundholders; and contract monitoring. To complicate matters further, by 1995 the Labour opposition was beginning to publish its strategy for the NHS and to indicate that general practice fundholders, under Labour, would be replaced by local commissioning teams and indeed that contracts would give way to rolling programmes of work (Labour Party 1995). Nevertheless, palliative care providers' worries about general practice fundholding continued to surface and concerns were again raised with the relevant minister about GPs' alleged lack of understanding of palliative care, the dangers of fragmenting services, and complications in payment arrangements (NCHSPCS 1996b). A talk on the 53 pilot schemes for total general practice purchasing, given to a national conference in 1996, revealed that only three of the schemes had stated palliative care as a priority, with 12 planning to purchase palliative or terminal care directly in 1996–7 (NCHSPCS 1996c). The following year a great deal of speculation about the impact of general practice fundholding and purchasing was brought to an end. The New Labour government produced its White Paper on the NHS and with it the statement that the schemes would cease.

One feature of the NHS and Community Care Act of 1991 was to throw into relief certain arbitrary distinctions between so-called 'health' and 'social' care. Whereas the former remained substantially free at the point of delivery, the latter was increasingly subjected to means testing. The arrangements were confusing for consumers of services and also led to 'cost shunting' between health and social services (Labour Party 1994). The Labour Party report on this issue was circulated with a press release drawing particular attention to the plight of terminally ill people discharged too early from hospital into nursing homes. The Conservative government's guidelines on the question of 'continuing care' had been published in early 1995 and included what it referred to as 'palliative health care' in the range of services which health authorities and general practice fundholders (where appropriate) must arrange to fund. Palliative health care could be taken to incorporate the following: in-patient palliative care in hospital or hospice and, in a limited number of cases, in nursing homes capable of providing this level of service, and specialist palliative care to people already in nursing homes, residential accommodation or in their own homes. However, it was acknowledged that priorities must be set within the total resources available – which would mean that the level of service could be expected to vary in different parts of the country. Health authorities were required to have their policies in place by April 1996 (Department of Health 1995). The view of the National Council for Hospice and Specialist Palliative Care Services was that terminally ill people should not be means tested, even where nursing home care or community care is required (NCHSPCS 1995d). Here was an example of government health policy – translated into a set of eligibility criteria for certain kinds of care – impacting directly upon the individual care of a very sick and dependent group of people. As on other occasions, however, policy debate could be turned to advantage and an increasingly well-organized palliative care lobby, through the National Council for Hospice and Specialist Palliative Care Services, was able to press the case for sensitive discharge procedures for those who may be within only days or weeks of death.

Just as the continuing care debate highlighted the inequitable distribution of long-term care services across the country, so too another major report of the period drew attention to persistent differences in the character and quality of one aspect of acute health care. In 1994 the Expert Advisory Group on Cancer published its findings first as a consultative document, then in final form in 1995, in what soon came to be known as the 'Calman-Hine Report' (Expert Advisory Group on Cancer 1995). The report was in part a response to what had come to be seen as the 'cancer lottery' – disparate outcomes of cancer treatment and care across the country and significant differences in survival rates between Britain and its European neighbours. A major restructuring of cancer services was proposed, comprising three tiers of organization in an integrated system encompassing primary care (for primary prevention, initial consultation and follow-up); cancer units (to treat the common cancers at district level); and cancer units (covering larger areas of population and dealing with rarer cancers and more complex problems).

Calman-Hine was seized upon by the palliative care community as an opportunity for development. Again, there was the potential to define the level of palliative care service appropriate for a given population. So for a population of 500,000, the following might be considered the norm: two full-time palliative care consultants; 25 specialist beds; twelve full-time clinical nurse specialists (two in hospitals, ten in the community); Marie Curie nursing for 50 per cent of all cancer patients at an average of 80 hours per patient; and 200 specialist palliative day care places per week. In turn the primary health care teams should develop a system to identify patients with cancer in their caseload; regular communication within the team about these patients; competence in basic symptom control; communication skills; criteria for referral to specialist palliative care; and improved interdisciplinary working. Within the cancer units it would be reasonable to find a specialist palliative care team with at least two full-time clinical nurse specialists and input from a consultant. In the cancer centres there should be teams with at least two such nurses and a full-time consultant (Oliver 1995). By late 1997, the impact of Calman-Hine was seen to have had the effect of raising the profile of cancer within the NHS. For Richards (1997) most effort appeared to have gone into the designation of cancer units (considered by many general hospitals to be essential to their survival). Less progress had been made at the primary care and cancer centre levels, though significant inequalities in the provision of specialist cancer services had been identified. Information flow and communication were highlighted as particular areas for development if primary care services, cancer site-specific teams and palliative care services were to combine to create a 'seamless service' (Richards 1997: 434).

We end this review of major health policy developments relating to hospice and palliative care over a 30-year period with some further observations on matters of finance and contracting for services. Such issues had affected the modern hospices from the outset. As the movement grew and as the NHS moved from a consensual model of administration to systems of prioritization based on management, and later market principles, so too the implications for palliative care became more complex. Throughout the middle years of the 1990s, therefore, as the Conservative reforms to the NHS took a hold, it was not surprising to see a careful watch being kept on questions of resource allocation and contracting.

As we have already seen, the ring-fencing of monies for independent hospices and for palliative care was dropped in 1995. Henceforth the monies disappeared into baseline budgets on a weighted capitation basis. Certain concerns persisted, especially in the independent hospice sector: small units had little potential for efficiency savings where most costs were taken up in salaries, and there was a need for purchasers to recognize the educational and training role of hospices (NCHSPCS 1994). However purchasers continued to be reminded by government circulars of their obligation to ensure that locally identified health needs for palliative care were being met. At the same time their difficulties in achieving this were evidenced in the lack of movement towards a 50–50 funding partnership between the NHS and the independent providers. Various studies showed that the government's contribution continued to hover at around 38 per cent of costs (Clark *et al.* 1997b) and this was a point which frequently arose in discussions between the National Council for Specialist Hospice and Palliative Care Services and ministers.

The activities of the National Council in these years did a great deal to raise the profile of palliative care among purchasers. In 1995 the Council embarked upon a strategy to influence purchasers. It produced a briefing pack of papers containing information about specialist palliative care services, outcome measures in palliative care and the needs of ethnic minorities. It also undertook, through its members, individual visits to three-quarters of all purchasing authorities in England and Wales (NCHSPCS 1997b). In addition it drew attention to the way in which general practice purchasing arrangements were being transformed. The task of contacting key decision makers in 109 health authorities was a significant one; but how to influence over 500 locality purchasing groups formed by coalitions between general practice fundholders? A review of the National Council's publications and activities in this period suggests however that, without its contribution, knowledge levels about palliative care among purchasers would have been considerably impoverished. Likewise and conversely, palliative care providers, guided by the Council's endeavours, undoubtedly became more sophisticated about policy matters and more aware of the changing implications of government thinking for their own area of work.

Between 1967 and 1997 palliative care in the United Kingdom passed from cautious beginnings to an increasingly emboldened period of expansion. Its ability to do this appears predicated on a growing willingness to work with the grain of government health and social policy. The early hospice founders had from the outset adopted a pragmatic approach to the NHS, sensing that they might not survive without cordial co-relations. As strategic planning became a more predominant part of the NHS culture of the 1970s, coexistence seemed ever more important: it would be unrealistic for hospices to imagine that they could pursue an isolationist course and also survive. At the dawn of the Conservative reforms of the 1990s the position was crystallized completely: join the contract culture or be condemned to obscurity. The independent hospices, after the briefest of vacillations, climbed on board and rarely looked back. Indeed there was even a sense of a certain elective affinity between the new business ethos of the NHS and that of the hospices. For the latter had now appointed their own chief executives, had adopted new strategies for income generation and fund-raising, and had taken on much of the corporate mantle of the Thatcher years. There we must pause our analysis, for the Thatcherite project, after briefly passing into the hands of a successor, eventually ran its course and ended in electoral disarray on 1 May 1997. In our final chapter we shall turn to the implications for palliative care of policy changes taking place under a New Labour government. Before that however we move our discussion of policy from the realm of macro changes in the NHS to an appraisal of the way in which individual palliative care services have been developing in community and in-patient settings of various kinds.

8 The delivery of palliative care services

In this chapter we now turn our attention to an examination of the current picture of palliative care delivery, and evidence from recent research about the effectiveness of different forms of delivery in meeting palliative care needs. Palliative care is multidisciplinary, involving the expertise of a variety of specialist and non-specialist staff. Further, its provision crosses institutional boundaries and the division between health and social care. This chapter gives some sense of the breadth of palliative care provision, and draws particular attention to how palliative care is perceived by patients and their informal carers, as well as by the professional staff responsible for care delivery.

The latest statistics available reveal the extent of proliferation, pluralization and 'partnership' within hospice and palliative care. We can see from Figure 4.1 that all forms of palliative care delivery have grown rapidly since 1965, but that home support has grown most significantly. Hospital-based palliative care has seen a sharp upturn since the mid-1980s when palliative medicine became a recognized specialty; while the provision of day care services now outstrips in-patient hospice provision.

Palliative care is delivered in various forms in all areas of the UK, although as we have seen, the growth of services has often been a piecemeal response to various influences such as local interest and the availability of charitable funding (Higginson 1997), rather than a planned response to guidance from government, although this is now a statutory requirement placed upon health authorities (Department of Health 1987).

Some 53,000 patient admissions to these services were recorded during 1993 (Eve and Smith 1996). While many services have coterminous organizational boundaries, with in-patient services in hospices and hospitals organizing both domiciliary outreach care and day care provision, we will discuss each form of provision as a separate entity for ease of presentation.

Hospital-based palliative care

Hospital palliative care teams (HPCTs) were pioneered in the UK at St Thomas's Hospital in 1976 (NCHSPCS 1996a). Their subsequent development was given impetus by DHSS guidelines published in 1987 which highlighted the need for an integration of care delivery for patients with palliative care needs. As we have seen, this formal adoption of palliative care stemmed largely from growing public recognition for the hospice movement, but it was also prompted by a tradition of research which highlighted the inadequacies of hospital care for dying people. For example, Wilkes (1984) had found that over 50 per cent of junior doctors and nurses felt that their training in terminal care was inadequate and most nurses described wards as unsuitable places to care for dying people. Wilkes's findings were supported by other researchers at this time. A particular problem highlighted was a lack of willingness on the part of clinical staff to disclose information about serious and terminal illness to patients (McIntosh 1977; Hinton 1980) and a lack of knowledge about pain and symptom control (Lunt and Hillier 1981; Hockley 1989).

Figures published by the National Council for Hospice and Specialist Palliative Care Services (1996a) show that between 1982 and 1996, the numbers of hospitals with either a multidisciplinary palliative care team or a palliative care clinical nurse specialist grew from five to 275. While these figures indicate an impressive rate of growth, it must be acknowledged that in the majority of cases (173 out of 275) hospital-based palliative care is the responsibility of one or two nurse specialists rather than a multidisciplinary team. Evidence about the difficulties faced by specialist nurses working alone and in a position of responsibility for altering traditional modes of service delivery may be found in the SUPPORT study commentary (SUPPORT Project Principal Investigators 1995) and in the report by Addington-Hall *et al.* of a randomized controlled trial of the effects of coordinating care for terminally ill cancer patients (Addington-Hall *et al.* 1992). In both of these studies a nursing intervention was designed to try to improve the coordination of care for dying people, but with little success. Difficulties were experienced particularly in exerting influence over the medical culture within which nurses had to work.

While some HPCTs have developed from existing symptom control or pain control teams, others have been initiated by pre-existing hospice services. Macmillan Cancer Relief has been a central player in the rapid growth of hospital-based palliative care, providing funds across a three-year period to give a firm foundation to new posts. This security has undoubtedly been important for the early success of posts, which may, by some hospitals, be considered unusual, innovative, and of questionable value. 'Pump priming' of NHS posts by means of charitable finance is a clear example of the

Figure 8.1 Levels of intervention by Hospital Palliative Care Team, Wellhouse NHS Trust 1995

Level 1	Advice and information may be accessed by professional colleagues directly with the team. No contact with the patient will be made by the team
Level 2	The team may make a consultative visit, preferably jointly with the referrer. Such visits will be single, unless requested otherwise by the referrer, and further contact will be made with the professional referrer only
Level 3	The team may make short-term interventions with the patient or family when specific problems need several visits. The intention is then to withdraw. Further referral may be made as necessary
Level 4	Ongoing, multiple-problem situations requiring continuing, regular assessment.

Source: Caddow, P., cited in NCHSPCS 1996a: 12

increasingly close relationship between the charitable and statutory sectors in palliative care delivery.

Some HPCTs have designated beds within the hospital for patients with palliative care needs. The presence of such beds is associated with the appointment of a consultant in palliative medicine to whom other hospital consultants can refer patients. More commonly however HPCTs take on an advisory role, acting as a specialist resource for the ward-based team or medical 'firm' which retains overall responsibility for the patient and family. In some cases HPCTs work within a hospital but have close professional and organizational links to a local hospice or community-based specialist service. The levels of intervention made by HPCTs will vary partly as a response to the constraints of these different organizational and professional contexts, but also in response to the more obvious factors of patient need and the knowledge of other health care professionals about palliative care. The National Council for Hospice and Specialist Palliative Care Services has published four levels of intervention based on those identified by Wellhouse NHS Trust symptom control team (NCHSPCS 1996a) (Figure 8.1).

The general responsibilities of HPCTs are also described, as the provision of

. . . emotional, psychosocial and practical support and symptom control to the patients and their family carers. This will often include the provision of additional information about diagnosis, progress and outcome of illness and help in making informed choices about future care and the circumstances of death ... An important aspect of the team's supportive role is promoting continuity of care from diagnosis through bereavement ...

                                                        (NCHSPCS 1996a: 12)

An insight into the practical execution of these very wide responsibilities and the extent to which they can be achieved can be gained from studying published accounts of the day-to-day operation of HPCTs. Kite's (1997) review gives a comprehensive overview of the range of research in this field. Here, we select a few examples for discussion.

George and Sykes (1997) give a detailed description of a service with a generic caseload. They describe how a potentially huge and varied workload is managed by the provision of focused support and consultation to other clinical teams. This may involve giving advice about an ethical dilemma, or may involve giving help in managing the terminal care of a person admitted as an emergency and found to be in the final stages of a chronic lung disease. The need for flexibility and for the adoption of a non-judgemental stance regarding the work and attitudes of non-specialist palliative care colleagues is highlighted in George and Sykes's account. For example, they describe how the demonstration of the effectiveness of palliative care in a broad range of clinical situations '... builds bridges, enriches hospital practice and restores the art of medicine' (1997: 246).

George and Sykes's observations and thoughts about the value of supportive collaboration are supported by Kite's (1997) review of models of care for dying people in hospital environments. Kite notes that by '... working alongside other hospital staff there are opportunities to share and disseminate palliative care skills widely, without deskilling those working in other specialities' (1997: 122). However Kite also points to the difficulties associated with the operation of HPCTs, namely the demanding nature of shared care and the difficulties of evaluating their effectiveness. Such concerns are clearly present in Hockley's account of the history and operation of an HPCT in Edinburgh (Hockley 1996).

Hockley describes how the palliative care team at the Western General Hospital, Edinburgh was established in 1993 following a review of care given to dying patients. The Directorate of Oncology then took the initiative to find charitable funding for a nurse specialist post. Two nurse specialists are now in post supported by consultants from two local hospices and, more recently, a specialist social worker. Hockley emphasizes the importance of having a permanent medical presence on the team. Such posts, she argues, give credibility to palliative medicine as a specialty and enable the palliative care aspects of an individual's care to be given a higher profile in the planning of appropriate medical treatment. The service is based in the Oncology Directorate but has the remit to serve the whole hospital. The effectiveness of the team has been assessed indirectly, first by reference to the steadily increasing number of referrals and second, by the decline in the number of complaints from relatives concerning the care of dying patients. Hockley describes in some detail the difficulties of running such a service:

> It takes time for a new service to become properly established and such a process has to be done gradually. There is no doubt that one can run the danger of being too idealistic about what can be achieved, especially if one's previous work has been within an isolated hospice setting. There is a danger in trying to be all things to all people in the acute setting especially if one is working on one's own before the establishment of the complete team . . .
>
> (Hockley 1996: 79)

Hockley emphasizes that acceptance of the need and value of an HPCT will be gradual. She implies that there may be resentment from other teams involved in patient care who may perceive an unnecessary duplication of their own skills, a detraction from their own skills or merely a 'hand-holding, second-rate, soft-option' (Kearney 1991 cited in Hockley 1996: 79).

Many hospital palliative care teams coordinate complex and highly integrated services which cross institutional boundaries. O'Neill *et al.* (1992) describe three such teams, based in the USA, UK and Canada respectively. In the UK example, in-patient care within the hospital is complemented by home care visiting services, an outpatient clinic and day care facilities. Staff work in adjacent offices which facilitates team working and coordination of care within the different settings.

Other researchers support the observation of O'Neill *et al.* that HPCTs may facilitate better links between hospital and home care. Bennett and Corcoran (1994) found that a hospital team working in Leeds increased significantly the number of referrals to palliative care services based in the community. Similarly, in a study of the impact of an HPCT on the care of 125 patients suffering from malignant disease, Ellershaw *et al.* (1995) found that 'appropriate' placements were facilitated by the formation of the team recording a discharge rate of almost 70 per cent of patients to other forms of care. Ellershaw *et al.* developed an assessment tool during the conduct of their study that indicated that distressing symptoms experienced by patients were significantly relieved. This latter finding echoes the results of McQuillan *et al.* (1996) who demonstrated that the introduction of an HPCT resulted in a significant increase in the use of opioid analgesics and non-steroidal anti-inflammatory drugs, and better symptom control among a group of patients with HIV-related disease and cancer.

Clearly the introduction of HPCTs can enhance the quality of care for those patients referred to their services. However, it is perhaps timely to reflect at this point that the vast majority of patients with palliative care needs within the hospital environment do not gain access to such specialized 'five star' management (Field 1994: 64). We saw in Chapter 5 that old people and people suffering from non-cancer disease fall most frequently into a position of acute disadvantage vis-à-vis palliative care provision. We have already examined some work of broad significance to this issue; here we introduce some more studies conducted in the UK.

In an observational study, Mills *et al.* (1994) describe the predominantly poor quality of care given to 50 dying patients in four teaching hospitals in the West of Scotland during the early 1980s. The study can be criticized for ethical shortcomings: for example, the authors report that they observed a patient who was in distress because of thirst, but they did not intervene in her care for some four hours. Further, it has been argued that there has probably been a marked improvement in the standards of care since the 1980s (Bennett *et al.* 1994; Stevenson 1994; Stone *et al.* 1994). These latter arguments are, however, based on largely unsubstantiated presumptions about the wide influence of palliative care support teams, and an expectation that attitudes and abilities to care have changed as a result of published policy guidelines on palliative care. Mills *et al.* present short case studies from 13 wards which highlight poor practices ranging from staff apparently failing to notice that someone had died, to a lack of attention to basic hygiene needs and a failure to provide oral fluids. During observations of ward rounds, Mills *et al.* describe how four 'caring' consultants paid attention to the 'holistic' needs of patients, while the remaining 19 apparently preferred to concentrate on the patient's disease and the relief of individual symptoms. Personal contact between patients and this latter group of consultants was minimal and became even less as death approached. A similar categorization was noted with regard to senior nurses. Three of the seven nurses observed presented the needs of patients to their medical colleagues and were persistent in their attempts to gain redress for those needs. The other four nurses did not introduce any aspect of patient care independently into the medical assessment of patients.

Although the tone of Mills *et al.*'s report is pessimistic, indeed shocking, they note that the general picture of poor care threw into

> . . . sharp focus the small group of senior medical and nursing staff who took time to be with the patient and who could be identified as carers by the attention to personal rather than technical matters. They identified all the needs of the person who was dying, explored various ways to give comfort and initiated medical and nursing measures to provide relief.
>
> (Mills *et al.* 1994: 585)

Mills *et al.* observe that there was a constellation of educational, environmental, financial and psychological constraints which combined to create the conditions in which the care that dying people received was frequently 'less than adequate'. Such observations of the critical influence of a range of external factors on the delivery of care to dying people are confirmed by Field's (1989) study of nursing in a general hospital and by other comprehensive accounts of the social context of care delivery in both hospital and community settings (Copp and Dunn 1993; Field and James 1993; James and Field 1996). Field's study is particularly illuminating however, since he shows that the palliative care approach may be delivered very effectively in one of the most highly technical areas of the hospital: the coronary care unit. His observations are supported by the recently completed research conducted by one of us (Seymour 1997) which demonstrated the care and compassion with which intensive care nurses approach dying patients and their families.

Other authors note similarly the possibility of developing a palliative care philosophy in acute hospital environments. For example, Haigh (1990) describes the successful introduction of a 'hospice ethic' into the nursing care of dying patients on a busy orthopaedic and trauma ward. This intervention reduced the isolation of dying patients by encouraging a culture that enabled nurses to sit with patients and enhanced links with the wider multidisciplinary team.

We conclude this section by referring to a valuable recent contribution to knowledge about the comparative value of hospital and hospice care. Seale and Kelly (1997) report a detailed analysis of comparative data on the care of 66 people who had died either in St Christopher's Hospice, London, or in nearby hospitals. This work was undertaken to enable comparisons to be made with earlier studies of the same settings which were carried out by Murray Parkes in 1967–9 and 1977–9 (Murray Parkes 1979a, b; Murray Parkes and Parkes 1984). The results suggest that in terms of symptom control hospital care has moved towards the standards of hospice care, but other key deficiencies remain:

> . . . this study reveals that the hospitals concerned still have some way to go in improving communication skills and the psychosocial climate, in spite of the provision of palliative care support terms in all the hospitals in the study. Hospital staff are still more likely to be seen as busy and the hospital atmosphere less 'like a family'. Large, mixed sex wards can be experienced as noisy, public places by the seriously ill and their families.
>
> (Seale and Kelly 1997: 98)

Palliative care at home

Although evidence suggests that most people would prefer to die at home, the numbers who actually achieve this wish are small. Increasingly, people with palliative care needs spend most of their last year of life at home with a final admission to hospital in the days immediately preceding death

(Townsend *et al.* 1990; Seale and Cartwright 1994; Addington-Hall and McCarthy 1995). In a prospective study of randomly selected patients with cancer from hospital and community settings who were expected to die within a year, Townsend *et al.* (1990) report that 67 per cent (41) of patients stated a preference to remain at home if their illness became worse, and if 'circumstances were instituted to allow the choice' (1990: 416). This compared to 16 per cent (10) of patients who said they preferred to die in hospital, and 15 per cent (9) who said they preferred hospice care. Significantly, Townsend *et al.* report that only 30 per cent (18) of patients actually died at home; and that of the 55 per cent (32) patients who eventually died in hospital, 82 per cent would 'ideally have preferred to die elsewhere'.

A range of constraints can prevent people from dying at home. In a review of the literature Hunt (1997) identifies haematological malignancy; disease of rapid progression; older age; low socio-economic status; and lack of access to palliative care services as variables which are associated with institutional death. Hunt further points out that cultural beliefs about the role of the family, and of the value of hospital care versus home care, will influence where people die (1997: 240). Most significantly, the degree to which palliative care needs can be met successfully in the home environment is shown to depend upon the close involvement and availability of an informal carer for the dying person: whether a family member or a close friend. The provision of adequate support for informal carers, together with appropriate medical and nursing interventions, appears to increase both the length of time that dying people remain in their own homes and the proportion of deaths that occur at home (Hunt 1997). As well as being most acceptable to patients and carers, the cost of home-based palliative care is significantly less than in-patient care. Thus in a discussion about the costs of different models of palliative care delivery, Whynes (1997: 36) notes that the setting in which care is provided at the end of life is '. . . a key determinant of overall costs'.

The provision of services and support at home to all dying people has been long recognized as a goal of health care policy. A recent illustration of this can be found in the recommendations of the Standing Medical Advisory and Standing Nursing and Midwifery Advisory Committees in 1992 (SMAC/SNMAC 1992), which took the view that all patients needing them should have access to palliative care services and that similar services should be developed for patients dying from diseases other than cancer. However, the evidence available currently reveals a picture of fragmentation of care delivery and a lack of 'fit' with patient and carer needs in the majority of cases. Clear inequalities of access to palliative care at home are present. Those with cancer are more likely to be offered the services of specialist home support services, moreover there are likely to be large variations in the provision of such services to cancer patients. In a survey of cancer deaths occurring during 1990, Addington-Hall and McCarthy

(1995) have shown that one-third of cancer sufferers either received no nursing care at all, although perceived by their informal carers as in need of care, or received insufficient nursing care. Less than one-third of cancer sufferers received care from Macmillan or hospice home care nurses.

For those suffering from non-cancer disease, palliative care is most likely to be delivered by primary health care teams, constituted by general practitioners, practice nurses and district nurses. The provision of specialist palliative care, whether at home, in a hospice or in hospital is extremely rare for this group of patients. Higginson (1997: 21) collates figures based on data collected by Addington-Hall and McCarthy (1995) which show, for example, that less than 1 per cent of 1622 patients with non-cancer disease were admitted to hospice care.

One of the most significant consequences of this inequality for the experience of dying is that those with non-malignant disease are less likely to have satisfactory symptom control, even when their symptom load is comparable to that suffered by cancer patients. In a comparative study of cancer and non-cancer patients Seale (1991a, c) found that surviving relatives of non-cancer patients reported that long-term pain, breathlessness and nausea were less well controlled. More recently, Skilbeck et al. (1997) found breathlessness to be a severe and unremitting problem for patients living at home with end stage chronic obstructive airways disease. General practitioners and community nurses recognize these shortcomings but express a lack of knowledge, time and nursing and medical resources for dealing with them (Seale 1992; Easthaugh 1996). While lack of symptom control is clearly a major factor involved in the experience of dying for the patients themselves, it also is highly likely to contribute to the experience of extreme stress among their informal caregivers. This has been found to be one mechanism which results in the emergency admission of dying people to hospital during the last week of their lives (Thorpe 1993).

Home-based palliative care is delivered by a wide variety of specialist and generic services, depending on local service availability, the condition from which the patient is suffering, the extent of his or her informal support, the patient's age and geographical location. We will discuss the main features of each type of service below, although readers will appreciate that services are not delivered on the basis of exclusivity: rather an individual may receive help from a number of different sources at any one time and at different points throughout his or her illness.

Primary health care teams

Primary health care teams are the first point of contact with health care for everyone living at home. The team usually consists of a general practitioner, a practice nurse and a district nurse. Each GP has a list of patients of between 1500 and 3000 (Doyle 1993: 629). It has been estimated that the average general practitioner will encounter only two patients per annum in need of specialist palliative care (NCHSPCS 1995c), although many others will have generic palliative care needs. Robbins *et al.* (1996) conducted a study looking at the role GPs played in the care of cancer patients which suggested however that there are significant variations around this figure (Robbins 1998: 115).

Recent studies suggest that primary health care team members regard palliative care as a high priority and recognize their frontline position in being the most likely source of support and help for people with palliative care needs. The introduction of GP facilitators to coordinate palliative care education in primary health care teams – a scheme introduced initially as a pilot in five areas in a collaborative project between the Royal College of General Practitioners and Cancer Relief Macmillan (1995) – reflects this concern very clearly. However, there is evidence which suggests that GPs experience significant difficulties associated not only with lack of specialist knowledge but also with lack of support from, and communication with, hospital specialists and other support services (Haines and Booroff 1986; Blyth 1990; Seale and Cartwright 1994; Addington-Hall and McCarthy 1995; Easthaugh 1996).

Studies of patients and informal carers' views of the primary health care team's role in delivering palliative care suggest that a pattern of general satisfaction with overall care by PHCTs is underpinned by specific concerns about communication, symptom control and carer support. In a significant number of cases in some areas however, the overall standard of care delivered by PHCTs has been reported as poor or very bad. For example, in a study by Higginson *et al.* of 65 patients and their carers in inner London and north Kent, 16 per cent of respondents in inner London fell into this category of response (Higginson *et al.* 1990). The authors suggest that this dissatisfaction may be related to '. . . a greater number of single handed general practices, a greater use of deputising services, difficulties in recruiting district nurses, and lack of commitment to co-ordinated care' (1990: 280).

Jones *et al.* (1993) conducted semi-structured interviews with 207 carers of deceased cancer patients in a more rural area, and report that in the vast majority of cases care was provided exclusively by the PHCT. Carers reported that while pain was well controlled, other symptoms were poorly controlled. Nursing care was perceived as insufficient by most of the carers involved in the daily care of the dying person:

> Practical nursing support was also lacking for most of the carers involved in daily care. Carers recalled feeling useless and helpless because they were not taught what to do.
>
> (Jones *et al.* 1993: 250)

Further, carers felt that their own needs were underestimated and that information about financial help and social service support was lacking.

While evidence about symptom control needs to be examined critically, since comparative research suggests that carers may either over- or under-estimate the degree of distress suffered by patients (Higginson *et al.* 1990; Hinton 1996), these findings are representative of those indicated in the small number of other studies which give information about user percep-tions of PHCTs (Sykes *et al.* 1992; Cowley 1993; McCarthy *et al.* 1997).

Other generic support services

Although people living at home with palliative care needs receive most of their care from members of their primary health care team, they will often be in receipt of some care from a wide range of other health and social service agencies, both statutory and voluntary. Social services may include home care workers; meals on wheels; social workers; laundry and incontin-ence services. Health services may include physiotherapy or chiropody, and visits from specialist staff from other clinical specialties such as stoma care or breast care nurses. Volunteers from local support groups may be available to help with respite sitting and bereavement follow-up or with social care needs such as shopping. The use of such support services may make a considerable difference to the quality of life for people with palli-ative care needs, helping them to maintain some independence and helping their families to care for them over a long period of time. However, their availability is very variable in different areas of the country and they are used by a minority of people with palliative care needs. Neale (1993: 12) in a study of informal palliative care in Newark notes that the primary health care team was the mainstay of support for families caring for people with palliative care needs, with only a 'small minority' receiving help from any other professional or voluntary source, even when care was known to be available.

The reasons for such limited uptake seem to be related to several factors. Clearly, some social support services such as home helps and meals on wheels are now subject to means testing; this may deter many people from making more use of them. Another factor may be related to a lack of knowledge about service availability and the process of applying for such help. More fundamentally, it may be that some forms of support services make little difference to the relief of the social and practical aspects of palliative care needs (Neale 1993; C.L. Clarke 1995). Lastly, research in the allocation of carer support shows that people living at home with a carer are often disadvantaged in terms of care provision, with those living alone most often in receipt of support (Qureshi and Walker 1989; Twigg *et al.* 1990). Neale's interview data from informal carers of people with palliative care needs capture what this means in terms of daily life:

> Well there was nobody else to care . . . it's a full time job . . . he's a bit incontinent right now. I've done two lots of laundry this morning . . .

and we've no washer... if he wants anything I do it straight away. That's why I don't do any house work ... I cut out all jobs as much as I can ... we have a home help but it's laughable. We've had her ten weeks now and she's been three times ...

(Neale 1993:16)

Research into the needs of people with HIV and their informal carers suggests, in keeping with research into other degenerative conditions such as dementia, that the course of illness is becoming of an increasingly unpredictable and chronic nature. Sufferers may require long-term 'packages' of care involving health, social and voluntary services (Handyside 1995). Successful, flexible and needs-led care delivery, however, requires a high level of ongoing collaboration between service providers. This may be difficult to achieve given the differences in ideology and institutional identification that exist among a wide range of providers (Layzell and McCarthy 1993). 'Cost shunting', identified recently as a problem in care of older ill people and in which individuals are passed between health and social care agencies, may also begin to feature in the care of people with HIV-related illnesses as the trajectory of deterioration lengthens and becomes uncertain. Similar problems have been identified in the care of people with chronic obstructive airways disease (COAD) and with chronic heart disease. For example, in a study of people with COAD, Skilbeck *et al.* (1997) report high levels of social isolation at home and a lack of strategic planning for care delivery at home. Individuals suffering from chronic obstructive airways disease had significant social, emotional, psychological, and information needs that were neither assessed consistently nor addressed adequately.

Specialist palliative care domiciliary services

In practice the boundaries between specialist palliative care home care teams and hospital palliative care teams are blurred. Often they are delivered from the same administrative centre and by staff who share responsibility for both types of service. Specialist palliative care teams that deliver services to people living at home may operate from a hospice, a hospital or a community unit, or be independent (Higginson 1997). They may deliver services to adults and children, or may be targeted specifically to serve the needs of children and their parents. Hockley (1997: 89–90) provides a clear account of respite at home teams, which are attached to hospices and which employ specially trained hospice nurses on a flexible 'nurse bank' basis.

Macmillan Nurses, who have a supportive and counselling role, may work as part of a specialist team including medical and social work staff, or work in isolation from others. Similarly Marie Curie Nurses, who provide practical nursing care, usually work alone. Marie Curie Nurses often do not have specialist training in palliative care (Higginson 1997), whereas

Macmillan Nurses are clinical nurse specialists in palliative care. Both Macmillan and Marie Curie Nurses may be funded partly by their respective charities and partly by health authorities or NHS trusts. A recent development in specialist services has been the introduction of Macmillan Carer schemes. These were introduced by Macmillan Cancer Relief in 1995 to provide support at home to patients and carers with palliative care needs. Key workers are specially trained health care assistants who provide for a range of health and social care needs (Ferguson *et al.* 1998).

Eve *et al.* (1997) identified 347 home care services operating in 1995. These services delivered care to an estimated 120,000 patients during 1995, of whom 65,000 died while receiving care from the teams and approximately 15,000 were discharged. 96.3 per cent of patients receiving care suffered from cancer and usually received care for between two and three months. Addington-Hall and McCarthy (1995) found in their survey that 29 per cent of people suffering from cancer in 1990 were in receipt of services from home care providers. Eve *et al.* (1997) estimate on the basis of their data that this figure is likely to have increased significantly during the last few years.

The majority of referrals for specialist palliative home care come from general practitioners (Eve *et al.* 1997). However, in a survey designed to elicit general practitioners' reasons for referral in Southampton, Pugh (1996) demonstrated huge variation in referral patterns according to individual GPs' working practices and beliefs about the value of specialist home care. Some GPs used services very frequently, while others never referred patients, preferring to manage their care alone or by making use of hospital services. The commonest reason for non-referral was that a patient's informal carer was 'coping well'. Further, some GPs seemed reluctant to share care with others. Finally, GPs had a perception that 24-hour cover and the provision of practical nursing by specialist staff was inadequate. This may have dissuaded some GPs from making better use of specialist services.

Boyd (1995a) points out that earlier studies indicated that specialist home care services sometimes lacked clear objectives and management, had little medical support and had difficult relationships with members of the primary health care team (Ward 1987; Lunt and Yardley 1988). These are difficulties which continue to be problematic although more recent evidence suggests that problems of role overlap, responsibilities for patient care and collaboration have begun to improve (Cartwright 1991; Boyd 1995b; Easthaugh 1996) and that specialist palliative home care teams have a recognized role in the home care of people with palliative care needs. Responsibility for out-of-hours care continues to be difficult to resolve, although Boyd (1995b) found that GPs express a willingness to share such 'twilight' care with specialist service providers.

Higginson *et al.* (1990) found that home care can significantly improve patient anxiety and symptom control, and improve communications between the patient and his or her informal carers. In a similar attempt to evaluate whether home care can achieve an acceptable quality of life for patients with terminal cancer and their carers, Hinton (1994) concludes that home care is largely successful in relieving distress and in promoting comfort, and that it avoids the high levels of pain and distress found previously in populations with no access to specialized home care:

> ... Brief distress was not – could not – be entirely avoided when severe physical symptoms or understandable feelings erupted. Distress demands help, and its persistence means help was unsuccessful or not offered. Although 15 per cent of these patients had physically distressed moments in the average week, only 2 per cent continued to be distressed for over 28 hours in that week ... Psychological distur-bance touched distress levels in 6 per cent each week, but persisted in only 1 per cent ...These data can be set against some recognised studies of terminal care such as Cartwright's sample of all deaths at all levels of care in England and Wales, in which relatives said that 69 per cent of patients had some distressing symptoms, and 42 per cent had pain.

(Hinton 1994: 195)

Hospice day care

Proponents of day care for people with palliative care needs argue that it is an important source of help with nursing and medical needs, and provides rehabilitation, social support and respite for patients and their carers (Fisher and McDaid 1996). Patients who have access to such services can spend more time at home than would otherwise be the case and may avoid full-time admission to hospice or hospital care. Sometimes day care centres are a 'stepping stone' to access to institutional care within the hospice to which they are usually attached (Lewis 1989). Further, it has been suggested that day care can provide a safe environment in which patients can begin to accept the enormity of a life-threatening illness and learn to live within its limitations (Hockley and Mowatt 1996). Reporting on early plans for a day care unit in Sheffield, Cockburn and Twine predicted a number of advantages over only providing in-patient beds:

> It would be possible for the discharged patients to return for at least one day a week to keep in touch and to receive support from the staff. It would also enable the early referrals to attend for day care and be supported as their illness progresses, so that they should be able to stay at home for longer.

(Cockburn and Twine 1982: 1410)

Recently, however, some doubt has been thrown on the value of day care as compared with other forms of service delivery. Indeed, the day care unit described by Cockburn and Twine at St Luke's Hospice, Sheffield, is facing imminent closure, with the suggestion that the palliative care needs for people living in the community are best met by services provided at home and by other agencies. Faulkner and Skilbeck (1995) conducted a survey of long-stay (one year and over) attenders in 125 hospice day care units, and report huge variation in the rates and length of patient attendance. Some units had as many as 27 long-term patients, and reported lengths of attendance of up to five years. Other units had much lower numbers of long-term patients who attended for periods of between one and five years. Such findings might suggest first, that day care provision is provided in an *ad hoc* and uncritical fashion to patients whose needs are not regularly assessed, and second, that day care hospices provide long-term social support which, although valuable, may be delivered at less cost by non-specialist services.

Figures from Eve *et al.* (1997) suggest that hospice day care is unequally distributed between men and women; old and young; and those suffering from cancer and non-cancer. Eve *et al.* (1997) show that hospice day care caters for more women than men, and that patients tend to be drawn from the older age groups, 65 years and over. These figures may reflect the fact that larger numbers of older women are more likely to live alone than men. It may also be the case that the communal and recreational activities provided by day care hospices are more attractive to women than men. Mirroring patterns of access to specialized home care services, day care provides over 96 per cent of its services to patients with cancer.

In-patient hospices

In-patient hospices are the original model of palliative care delivery, and as such have exerted a fundamental influence on patterns of palliative care provision in the UK. Hospices may be voluntary, meaning that they are an independent charity, or may be an NHS palliative care unit or centre. Voluntary hospices have developed close links with the NHS in terms of funding, contractual relationships, policy guidelines and staffing.

Some hospices provide a service exclusively for children, while others provide a service for people with HIV-related illnesses. Most, however, provide nursing and medical care for people with cancer and a small number of other conditions such as motor neurone disease. The 1997 hospice directory indicates that in January 1997 there were 223 in-patient hospices: 148 voluntary units, 11 Marie Curie Centres, 8 Sue Ryder Homes and 56 NHS managed units. Hospices now exist in all areas of the UK, although they remain slightly more concentrated in the South East of England as a consequence of an early proliferation in more affluent areas of the country.

Eve *et al.* (1997) show that 65 per cent of patients admitted to hospices during 1994–5 were over the age of 65. There was an almost equal distribution of men and women, but an under-representation of people from ethnic minority groups. Approximately 17.5 per cent of people who died from cancer during 1994–5 were cared for in a hospice. In the smaller units the mean length of patient stay was under 13 days, while patients admitted to the larger units had admissions of between 15 and 16 days. In some circumstances patients may stay in hospices for several weeks, while others are admitted for short periods of respite care and symptom management. Extrapolating from these statistics, Eve *et al.* suggest a number of possible, but as yet unsubstantiated, underlying trends:

> This may mean that patients admitted to the larger units are more ill and more dependent. It may be that, on the whole, the larger units lie in large cities and towns and admit more patients with overwhelming social needs from particularly deprived areas in their catchment. It may be that the problems of bed management are more acute and that there is consequently greater pressure to free a bed for a new admission. Clearly this is an area for more specific research than is possible from the data collected through this survey.
>
> (Eve *et al.* 1997: 40)

As Hockley points out (1997: 85), criteria of admission to in-patient hospices have always been an important issue. Criteria may well have to be tightened where beds are not easily available, and so obviously will vary with local demand for services, with unit size and with the availability of other forms of care. Admission is arranged by the senior nurse or doctor within each unit, following a referral from hospital or community services. The largest percentage of admissions come from patients at home (Eve *et al.* 1997; Hockley 1997).

Hospices are usually staffed by a combination of voluntary and paid workers; the latter may hold NHS contracts, rather than be the employees of the charity responsible for the management of the hospice. As Salisbury (1997: 48) points out, the philosophy of hospice care builds on that originally established at St Christopher's hospice and involves '. . . a personal non institutional approach, promoting psychological and physical well being through good symptom control. The whole person approach respects patients' autonomy and choices, and open communication is encouraged'. Detailed descriptions of hospice nursing and culture may be found in the ethnographic accounts of Hockley (1990) and James (1986). Hockley and James use ethnographic methods, principally participant observation, to give rich descriptions of the daily care of dying people. Hockley compares three settings: a hospice, a residential home and a community-based bereavement counselling service, while James focuses predominantly on 'carework' within the hospice environment. From their detailed accounts we are able to develop some sense of the 'life-world' of dying people within these various settings and can appreciate how the experience of dying is critically contingent on the style of social relationships with which they are surrounded.

Johnson *et al.* (1990) provide evidence of the range of activities in which hospices engage, based on a questionnaire survey which achieved a response from 85 per cent of in-patient units. The data collected suggest that there are wide variations in the type of care offered to patients. Some units place emphasis on the provision of terminal care, while others emphasize rehabilitation and short-term symptom control. Death and discharge rates per bed per year vary from 1.6 to 31.8 in different units, with throughput increased significantly in units where there was a full-time consultant or medical director. These units were also much more likely to undertake a range of clinical investigations and treatments, a finding confirmed by Ahmedzai *et al.* some six years later in a follow-up survey (Ahmedzai *et al.* 1996). These findings suggest that 'hospice' may not be as uniform an entity as its widely accepted, almost ideological, public image tends to imply. Johnson *et al.* argue that such figures

> . . . should dispel the continuing misconception among the public and some health professionals that the sole function of the hospice is to provide 'tender loving care' during the last few days of life. Not only are many patients discharged from (rather than die in) a hospice but our findings suggest that their management is likely to include a range of investigations and procedures that are usually associated with acute hospital care.
>
> (Johnson *et al.* 1990: 792)

The observations of Johnson *et al.* capture the ongoing debate about the meaning and place of hospice care in the care of seriously ill and dying people. As we discussed in Chapters 5 and 6, the tension between medicalization and demedicalization is a very real issue in hospice care, and has resulted in some polarized views about the proper purpose of such care (Ahmedzai 1993; Biswas 1993), and the extent to which hospice care is becoming reincorporated into mainstream medical and nursing provision.

One approach to the evaluation of hospice care has been to draw comparisons between hospice care and other forms of care. Seale and Kelly's research (1997) discussed above is one recent example of this, and other work of this kind is discussed at some length in Chapter 6. Comparative analysis in this way allows us to make some judgements about the ways in which hospice care is different, and how those who receive such care perceive it. All the evidence so far reviewed suggests that those who receive hospice care value it particularly for the 'human' approach it can offer, for the reductions in anxiety and improvements in communication it can achieve and for the standards and style of nursing care which it delivers

(Killbery 1997: 81). As indicated in Chapter 6 however, the diversification of 'hospice' and the movement of patients from one setting to another makes these differences difficult to establish, except in those cases that most clearly approximate to some traditional version of the hospice model.

A distinction needs to be drawn here, however, between the needs and wants of *individuals* and the needs and wants of *population*. What may deliver an excellent standard of care to a small group of individuals and their informal carers may not contribute much to the practical relief of palliative care needs in the wider community. Other forms of care may be both more effective and more equitable in meeting the palliative care needs of the whole population. A recent review of the costs and benefits of different models of palliative care (Bosanquet *et al.* 1997) suggests that little cross-comparative research has been conducted on different forms of care in the UK, although evidence from the USA suggests that home-based care is more acceptable to both patients and carers, less costly and more equitably distributed than institutional hospice care. In the UK, the emphasis has been on the collection and evaluation of evidence to improve care within units, rather than a critical analysis of the continued benefits of in-patient hospice provision.

Institutional homes for older people

For the group of people most likely to die (the very elderly), care before death tends to be given within residential and nursing homes. There has been a huge proliferation of private homes during the last decade, encouraged by reform of financial arrangements for long-term care, and the reduction in the availability of NHS beds for very old people. Approximately 50 per cent of all people aged 85 years and over live in residential and nursing homes and 15 per cent of all deaths now occur within their walls (Bury and Holme 1991; Field and James 1993; Seale and Cartwright 1994). Women are more likely to receive institutional care than men, and data from Doncaster (Sims *et al.* 1997) suggest that older people from social classes IV and V are more likely to die in nursing and residential homes than people from any other social class. There is also significant geographical variation in the availability of institutional care (Sinclair 1988; Henwood 1990; Benzeval *et al.* 1995).

Nolan *et al.* note that the prospect of residential and nursing home care is a source of great anxiety for older people and their informal carers. This stems in part from the legacy of 'negative and dysfunctional image of institutional care' (1996: 127), but also reflects a realistic assessment of the limited extent of choice and control which can be achieved during the process of admission and during care delivery. Admission to institutional care usually occurs suddenly after hospital treatment for an acute exacerbation of chronic illness, and may signal the fundamental transformation of a long-term caring relationship between an old person and his or her close companion. The loss of co-residence and the centrality of the caring relationship have been identified as significant sources of grief and guilt (Lewis and Meredith 1989; Nolan *et al.* 1996), and may be exacerbated by a sense of exclusion from the activities of professional caregivers. Equally, admission to institutional care may appear inevitable when an old person who becomes ill has no informal carer readily available. Many family members live long distances from one another; this has been shown to contribute to the likelihood of institutional care when older persons become unable to care for themselves at home. The inner cities have been affected particularly by migration of younger family members, leaving a disproportionate number of older people in need of care and support from formal sources (Sinclair 1988; Joseph and Hallman 1998).

Older people living in institutional care are very likely to be suffering from a complex combination of chronic illnesses and to be significantly more physically and cognitively disabled than those living at home or with their families (Bury and Holme 1991; Field and James 1993; Seale and Cartwright 1994). Dementia is a particularly common cause of severe disability and a common cause of admission to institutional care (Levin *et al.* 1989). Those who are particularly frail and ill live predominantly in nursing homes where, as their title suggests, some trained nursing staff are available to give nursing care. In practice however, as Field and James (1993) note, the boundary between nursing home and residential home is blurred, with many people who require higher levels of support living in residential homes.

Clearly all institutional homes have an important role to play in meeting the palliative care needs of a significant proportion of older people. Hockey notes, for example, that the care of the sick and dying within the nursing home she studied was '... an intrinsic aspect of its role ... deterioration and death were always waiting in the wings' (1988: 201). However, standards and styles of care delivery within institutional care have always been, and continue to be, a source of concern both for professional commentators and for older people and their families (Townsend 1964; Booth 1985; Holmes and Johnson 1988; Phillips *et al.* 1988; Royal College of Nursing 1992; Seale and Cartwright 1994; Nolan *et al.* 1996). For example, a participant observation study of three residential homes highlighted the uniform, regular lives of residents, their marked social isolation and the over-burdened workloads of the care staff:

A few did go outside their homes, but even fewer had visitors. The life of the communal sitting room was the centre of the home and, where people had single rooms, they seemed to use them to shut out the world as far as possible . . . Contact seemed to be primarily associated with the daily tasks of physical care. This may of course involve emotional care, but it is difficult to imagine this as a frequent occurrence while the care assistant, faced with a heavy workload, was hurrying to put a resident on a commode, wheel him or her to breakfast, feed him or her custard by the spoonful, or sort out dirty washing . . . The one observation out of 219 of what might really be called emotional or pastoral care found the chef in one of our homes talking, in his spare time, to a resident who was bed bound and soon to die of cancer.

(Phillips *et al.* 1988: 89)

Studies of nursing homes raise identical concerns. Challis and Bartlett (1988) refer to their perception of an 'undercurrent of sadness' in the nursing homes they visited; while Holmes and Johnson documented detailed examples of grossly inadequate nursing care of residents and poor conditions and pay of care staff in private nursing homes (Holmes and Johnson 1988). More recently, the Royal College of Nursing has conducted a survey of nursing staff in nursing homes (1992), and describe the results as suggesting that care in homes is at best variable, and at worst, a 'scandal waiting to happen'. A heavy reliance on poorly paid unqualified care staff and a lack of opportunity for continuing education among qualified nursing staff (Gibbs 1995) clearly contributes to this situation.

Shemmings (1996) draws attention to cultural differences between institutional homes and hospices which may adversely affect the quality of life *and* death for residents. A key difference may be a general unwillingness among institutional care staff to discuss death and dying. This can create a situation in which any degree of choice and control over the manner of death is absent. Shemmings draws on early work by Hinton (1972) and Townsend (1964), as well as later studies, suggesting that

On entering residential care there is a covert understanding that elderly people will end their days there, and yet often it is not considered 'decent' to broach the subject of how they wish to be cared for when dying, and what services the home offers . . . Hinton (1972) observed further that there was a veil of silence in some residential homes. A game is thus devised, with its own unspoken rules and rituals . . .

(Shemmings 1996: 32)

Qualitative interviews with care staff in five homes conducted by Shemmings (1996) suggest a low level of emotional or educational readiness for caring for dying people. This manifested itself in various ways, but was particularly clear in expressions of feelings of 'helplessness' and of physical and emotional exhaustion (Shemmings 1996: 65–9).

We are awaiting currently the results of a three-year study into the management of death in residential and nursing homes (Komaromy 1995,

1997) which will shed further light on these issues. The focus of this work is to assess the extent to which hospice philosophy has permeated the culture of institutional care, and the extent of preparedness among staff to assume hospice-style care. Interim results (Komaromy 1995) suggest that care staff *do* wish to be able to care for residents until they die. Up-to-date evidence about their ability and resources to do so is eagerly awaited.

While variability in standards and quality of nursing care give rise to concern, responsibility for the medical treatment of residents is also problematic. General practitioners provide most of the medical care for residents, but many private homes are reluctant to pay for this service and many GPs are hard pressed to provide an adequate level of care (Cartwright 1991; Field and James 1993). The transfer of ill residents to hospitals and hospices may be one solution to this problem, but as Field and James note (1993: 20), those living in institutional homes are less likely to be transferred to other care settings than those living elsewhere. As a result, standards of pain and symptom control may be poor, with medication use both inappropriate and haphazard particularly in private homes (Sinclair 1988; Keay *et al.* 1997). Pain in older people has been shown to be under-recognized in acute hospital settings where trained staff are more readily available (Ahronheim 1997); it is highly likely therefore, that this is even more of a problem in settings where there is a lack of trained staff.

Some commentators argue that nursing homes must be regarded as providers of palliative care (Maddocks 1996). The epidemic of 'terminal suffering' (Ahmedzai 1995) experienced by older people suffering from dementia is evidence of the pressing need for institutional homes to recognize their role in palliative care delivery and be provided with the support to provide a good standard of care to their patients. The interest in palliative care may be seen as an encouraging sign that some homes are willing to take on this challenge, however the reality of their ability to provide holistically for the complex palliative care needs of their patients continues to be a source of concern. Maccabee (1994: 211) has argued that the 'constant demand on inpatient hospice services has led to an increasing use of nursing home beds for patients requiring longer-term nursing care . . . the transfer of a patient from a palliative care unit to a nursing home may lead to a shortfall in meeting the needs of patients and relatives'. The reasons underpinning this shortfall are currently not well understood but appear to be related to a number of features. First, institutional homes are not currently included in the educational activities promoted by palliative care organizations. Second, they continue to have poor links with other service providers. Third, their current reliance on poorly paid and untrained care assistants may be the fundamental barrier to the provision of skilled care necessary for the relief of palliative care need. Most fundamentally, the issues of resources and of who *pays* for good quality palliative care among older people in institutional care are the questions which require urgent

attention. Until these matters are resolved institutional homes will continue to share many of the features of poor palliative care provision that
were so prevalent in hospital practices of earlier decades and to which the
hospice movement was, in part, a response.

As we have seen contemporary palliative care spills over a number of
boundaries: institution and home; statutory and voluntary; day care and
in-patient care. We have examined each of these settings in some detail,
drawing extensively on a range of recent research to delineate their key
features and to identify how their services are perceived by those who
receive them and those who deliver them. It will be apparent however that
there is little evidence either about the movement of patients from one setting to another or about the kind of care that people with life-threatening
illness receive in settings where specialist palliative care is not available.
The official statistics relating to place of death are perhaps most illuminating. We have seen that hospice care actually provides for a tiny minority of
dying people. Most people spend the last year of their lives at home and
come into hospital in the few days immediately before death (Neale 1991;
Seale and Cartwright 1994). The majority of those who die at home
depend largely upon informal carers, usually a member of the immediate
family, backed up by general practitioner services. The provision of specialist
palliative care remains focused on those suffering from cancer rather than
from degenerative disease from other causes. Neale summarizes the position
in a review of informal palliative care needs, drawing on a broad range of
research:

> . . . it is clear that in future most patients will die in hospital, or at
> home without specialist support, rather than in a hospice. Recent
> research has revealed the plight of terminally ill patients and their
> families who have little choice over the setting and style of their care
> and death because their disease is non-malignant. Such families are
> rarely eligible for hospice care or specialist home or hospital support
> since these services are still provided almost exclusively for cancer
> patients . . . Moreover, it appears that only a minority of cancer pa-
> tients receive specialist support. Barnet and McCarthy (1986) who
> followed up the 75 per cent of cancer patients and their families who
> had *not* been referred to the support team prior to their discharge
> from hospital, found that while some were well cared for by the
> primarily health care team, others remained in severe difficulties, un-
> discovered by both GPs and hospital doctors.
>
> (Neale 1991: 22)

Coordination of care as patients and their families move between settings
and agencies at the end of life is clearly of paramount importance. Growing
policy concern with the role of primary care clearly implies that this is the
linchpin around which all other services should turn.

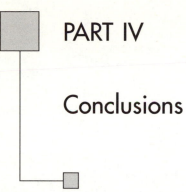

PART IV

Conclusions

Introduction to Part IV

We come to the end of our reflections on palliative care and face the anxiety-provoking task of reaching some conclusions. How best to construct these and how to seek some integration between the sociological, historical and policy perspectives from which we have viewed our subject matter? Perhaps unwisely, we have chosen to do this through that risky social science occupation of turning our attention to questions about the future.

We begin this by reiterating some of the conditions of late modernity as they apply to the experience of illness, disease and health care. We would never seek to underplay the tangible and obdurate properties of illness experience, but we also are persuaded that these take particular forms within the dispositions of late modernity. Illness, the body and the self are conjoined in ways that may well threaten the ontological security of those involved. Likewise in a culture which is frequently organized around a systematic amnesia about our mortality, the process of dying, even at the end of a long life, poses particular kinds of existential problems.

We try to suggest here that these points are not only relevant to sociological argument, but that they also have a bearing on how palliative care might develop in the future. Indeed, some of these features of individualism, consumerism and reflexivity are finding their way into questions of policy. Certainly one reading of the 1997 White Paper on the National Health Service, with its emphasis on 'partnerships', constellations of values and alliances, would confirm this. We therefore conclude with a plea for palliative care to embrace more actively such late modern dispositions; to become more reflexive; to widen its vision; to tackle new agendas; and to seek to promote its important principles and practices not only in the affluent nations, but all around the world.

9 The future for palliative care

In late modern culture new ways of talking about dying and death are emerging. In the prosperous, consuming societies of the affluent world at the beginning of the twenty-first century many paradoxes exist around the subject of human mortality. On the one hand, as Small puts it, 'we have decided that dying is what other people do' (1997b: 218). In other words there remains evidence of a secular, historical trend to repress matters of death and dying, to marginalize and stigmatize and to render death 'taboo'. Alternatively, as Walter argues, a 'revival of death' is underway which is 'increasingly being shaped by neither the dogmas of religion nor the institutional routines of medicine, but by dying, dead or bereaved individuals themselves' (1994: 2). We suspect that neither of these authors would disagree with each other's statements, preferring to recognize instead the potential for a variety of discourses to coexist, to compete and to countermand one another. Yet as many commentators have also highlighted, a further dimension of the contemporary culture of death requires consideration, and that is the extent to which it now attracts the attention of specialized practitioners, of professional and voluntary organizations, of empirical researchers and of social theorists. We would be fairly confident in asserting that much more is now being written and debated concerning aspects of death and dying than was the case 50 years ago: when it would, for example, have been impossible to have written this book. Our purpose here, of course, has not been to review all of these issues. Rather we have focused, perhaps narrowly, on a specific manifestation of contemporary deathways: the hospice and palliative care movement. Yet we have found within that single domain of enquiry much which is of sociological, historical and policy interest.

Let us first of all remind ourselves of the wider context in which hospice and palliative care have been developing. We have seen that social theorists continue to argue that death occupies an ambiguous position within late modern culture, in which it is simultaneously 'absent' and 'present'. So whilst the experience of dying is sequestrated in hospital wards and specialist institutions, other representations of death proliferate within newspapers, television, film and the Internet. At the same time late modern culture harbours profound and chronic doubts about 'knowledge', 'truth' and 'reality'. Our understanding of the world is therefore open to continuous revision, is temporary and 'just for the moment'. Similar processes are at play at the level of human identity; the self has become malleable as never before and 'who' we are becomes a reflexive project capable of sustained reworking and reformulation across what Frankenberg (1987) sees as the 'pilgrimage' of the life course. Accordingly, personal encounters with death may be experienced as fateful moments within the pilgrimage, when order gives way to disorder, structure to anti-structure, and formal association to a sense of what Victor Turner calls 'communitas' (Turner 1969). At such times our 'business as usual' orientation to life becomes unsustainable; we may come to see the world in new ways, to form new social relationships, to challenge prevailing norms and values.

Of course, death poses particular dilemmas in this regard. The biological facticity of death, once regarded as relatively unproblematic, has now come to represent a contested arena where medicine, ethics and the law frequently meet. Debates proliferate about what constitutes the state of death. This is consistent with another prevailing trait of late modernity: the prevalence of risk and uncertainty (Beck 1992). Here we see the propensity for individuals to assess a competing array of the 'risks' which may threaten their health, quality of life, indeed everything they take at face value. So it is that individuals, organizations and governments must become expert at strategies for risk management, in trading off the likely risks and rewards of a given situation and even, at times, in entering into risk situations for the perceived benefits which may subsequently derive.

This relates to our point in Chapter 1 about the moral order of suffering. The risk of suffering can be assessed at the individual, social and societal levels. Likewise matters of life and death, about sustaining or withdrawing treatment for the very ill, about easing death's pains or hastening its arrival, these constitute a risk terrain of judgements, decision making and practical action affecting patients, their associates, professionals and policy makers. The 'abstract systems' described by Giddens (1991) provide in a sense some shield of ontological security in the face of such manifold risks. By trusting to the expertise of others and to the wider systems in which they are located we are spared some of the doubts which 'knowing' might engender. In this sense, health care is a classic abstract system, constructed in its day-to-day workings to elicit our compliant and uncritical faith. Nevertheless, in late modern times even such abstract systems are vulnerable to a sense of doubt which pervades the contemporary attitude. As Turner (1996) puts it, there is a fluidity about medicine and science in post-modern culture and this heightens the sense of the body and self as uncertain projects: '... the modern self corresponds to and is produced by a new uncertainty, differentiation and fragmentation of the risk society' (Turner 1996: 21).

A great deal of sociological interest in embodiment began with Foucauldian notions of the body as the site of inscription by the disciplinary power of modern medicine (Foucault 1973). Crossley (1996) however draws attention to an important division which is forming in the social theory of the body. Within this division *the body as lived* is counterposed to *the body as inscribed*. The first position draws on a tradition emanating from the work of the French philosopher Maurice Merleau Ponty, and is phenomenological in character. In this framework, to be human is to belong to the world, and embodied action is identified with the production of meaning. The second position emanates from the work of Michel Foucault and sees the behaving body as subject to historical forms of conduct which not only mould the body, but also force the bearer of these conducts to accept responsibility for them. Helpfully, Crossley does not seek to collapse these two positions into a unified system but suggests that both are of relevance in understanding the problem of embodiment.

All of these ideas we find useful in making sense of palliative care from a wider, sociological perspective. In this final chapter therefore we wish to build on these insights as we explore a theme which has generated considerable commentary in recent times. We refer to the question of *the future for palliative care*.

We start this discussion from a position outlined by Bauman, which sees mortality as central to human culture and which, for us, opens up wider possibilities for thinking about how and why palliative care has emerged as a specific field, and where it might be heading:

> There would probably be no culture were humans unaware of their mortality ... Culture would be useless if not for the devouring need of forgetting; there would be no transcending were there nothing to be transcended.
>
> (Bauman 1992: 31)

By taking this wider view of the relationship of mortality to human culture we are perhaps able to see some aspects of the future of palliative care in a different light, and to generate broader conclusions.

Some propositions about the future for palliative care

Palliative care and society

Our first point should be obvious to anyone who has read the whole of this book, rather than simply skipped to the conclusion. Clearly, we subscribe to the view that any analysis of future developments in palliative care must pay attention to the wider sociological and historical context and must not be sidelined into narrow technical debates or interprofessional preoccupations. From this point of view, palliative care has to be seen as an aspect of culture through which the dilemmas of human mortality are being dealt with at a specific time. So it is important to keep in mind that palliative care arises in the context of religious pluralism; scepticism about medicine; health care consumerism; and reflexivity in the body and the self. In this sense palliative care has been engaged in the production of a new ethic of care for the dying which reflects late modern preoccupations. At the same time this viewpoint emphasizes the need for palliative care to itself become reflexive in orientation, more willing to take the position of the other (particularly on ethical matters relating to euthanasia), more ready to acknowledge its own weaknesses, its temporary and contingent status. Because of their history, this is something which British hospices may find particularly difficult and we are reminded of Abel's (1986) point that the American hospices encapsulated both revolutionary *and* conservative elements. Doyle alludes to a similar problem:

> Doctors and nurses in general hospitals, often working in inadequate surroundings with insufficient resources yet with the highest of ideals, have come to feel that they can never achieve the standards which they are led to believe are universal in palliative care units.
>
> (Doyle 1994: 380)

So in this sense palliative care can be seen in a dialectical relationship to the society in which it is located, and in relationship to the system of health and social care in particular. At the macro level of vision and aspirations, palliative care has the ability to reflect the preoccupations of late modern culture and to articulate these in a programme of action. At the meso – or micro – levels however, palliative care also has the potential to alienate those in cognate disciplines as it perpetuates and comes to believe in its own internally referential ideologies. Such factors could be crucial in shaping future directions.

Solution or manifestation?

Whilst it is therefore tempting to see palliative care as the *solution* to certain problems, it may be more helpful to regard it as a *manifestation* of them. Of course, the early hospice movement with its reformist, oppositional stance has worked hard to make claims for the transformation of contemporary deathways. Few would deny that hospices *have* made a major contribution to this; but we must also ask how it was that the hospice movement itself became possible. These conditions of possibility, we would argue, go beyond the existence of a small number of charismatic and highly-motivated individuals. Preferable then to see palliative care as part of the multifaceted tensions and contradictions surrounding the meaning of death in society itself. This in turn links to our first proposition – that if palliative care is to continue to develop it must remain alert to the detailed preoccupations of those who use its services. Of special relevance here is the situation of older people, which we have considered at various points in earlier chapters. The early decades of the twenty-first century will not only see major increases in the numbers of elderly people, but the make-up of that group will also become much more diverse, reflecting the range of ethnicities, social classes, sexual orientations and lifestyles within society. Tomorrow's older people will consequently have different ideas and expectations to those of a generation earlier and palliative care will need to be responsive to this.

Status ambiguity

Our third proposition is that palliative care as a set of activities and an emergent specialty is currently beset by status ambiguity, imprecise definition and uncertainty of mission. Much of the recent debate in the British context has focused around how palliative care should be defined. On the one hand Doyle can write: 'It is probably true to say that *palliative care, hospice care*, and *terminal care* are interchangeable terms all meaning one and the same thing' (Doyle 1994: 378) (italics in original).

Yet within a short period of time the National Council for Hospice and Specialist Palliative Care Services can establish a working party of experts to consider questions of definition and to promote the distinction between 'the palliative care approach', 'specialist palliative care' and 'palliative medicine' (NCHSPCS 1995c). Within this new lexicon 'terminal care' is seen as only a part of palliative care and the term 'hospice care' is quietly abandoned. Such attempts at clarity of definition are of course important and there may well be a growing consensus of understanding within palliative care as to what the definitions connote. At the same time even the term 'palliative care' appears to be not well understood by the general public and as one consultant in the discipline recently remarked at a conference, 'I belong to a specialty about which most of my colleagues in medicine haven't got a clue'. Of course, we also acknowledge that this is changing. A major breakthrough, for example, has been the requirement that health commissioners ensure that the 'palliative care approach' is being adopted across a wide range of local health care services for which they are responsble (National Health Service Executive 1996). But far greater clarity is required about what constitutes palliative care, not least on the part of those who provide it as their main area of work.

Policy influences on future developments

This brings us back to wider questions of policy which may shape the future of palliative care. In Chapter 7 we indicated that we would return to the latest manifestations of these by way of conclusion. As we write, many stakeholders within the UK palliative care arena are beginning to speculate on the likely impact of the New Labour government's White Paper on the health service (Department of Health 1997). Here we summarize briefly the changes proposed in the White Paper and offer some early thoughts on its implications for palliative care.

Many have welcomed the 1997 White Paper for its focus not only on ill health but also for its recognition of the persisting problem of inequalities in health. This is done in the context of some major long-term challenges to the delivery of any health care system: growing public expectations; the spectre of rationing versus unaffordable levels of funding; medical advances; and demographic changes, particularly relating to older people. Six key principles are identified:

- To renew the NHS as a genuinely *national* service.
- To make the delivery of health care a matter of *local* responsibility within a framework of *national* standards.
- To develop NHS *partnerships*, especially with local authorities.
- To improve *efficiency* by a more rigorous approach to performance and by cutting bureaucracy.
- To shift the focus onto the *quality* of care and to promote *excellence*.
- To rebuild public *confidence* in the NHS.

(Department of Health 1997: 11)

Certain elements of earlier reforms, including of course those of the predecessor Conservative government, are retained in the 1997 White Paper. Seen as 'keeping what works' (1997: 11), these include the separation of the planning of hospital care and its provision; the growing centrality of primary care; and decentralized responsibility for operational management through NHS trusts. A clear and continuing commitment to health needs assessment is also discernible. At the same time, there is an emphasis on 'discarding what has failed' (1997: 12). Chiefly included here is the abolition of the internal market as a 'misconceived attempt to tackle the pressures facing the NHS' (1997: 12). Criticized specifically are fragmentation and lack of coordination and the unfairness of the market system, together with the bureaucratic distortions and secrecy which it generates. In particular, general practice fundholding (which, as we have seen, has caused so much anxiety for palliative care providers) is brought to an end by the White Paper.

So what new recommendations are proposed? These are most visible in the sphere of primary care. In England 500 'primary care groups' consisting of GPs and community nurses, with an average catchment of 100,000, are to be established (in Scotland primary care trusts will be formed). The primary care groups will take on a wide range of commissioning tasks and their governing bodies will include social services representatives in a bid to foster greater integration between health and social care. Also proposed is a reduction in the number of health authorities, whose role will shift towards the development of Health Improvement Programmes; working with primary care groups, social services, hospital trusts and other agencies, they will take on a more strategic role and relinquish their 'commissioning' functions. Some pooling of budgets between health and social services will take place and annual NHS contracts will be replaced by three-year agreements. Health Improvement Programmes will focus on the most important health needs of the local population and Health Action Zones (begun in April 1998) will give attention to areas of extreme health need. At the same time there will be a strong commitment to addressing the problem of variable clinical standards across the country through the creation of National Service Frameworks and a National Institute for Clinical Excellence. These will monitor, respectively, equity of access and standards of care (taking a cue from the Calman-Hine reforms we discussed in Chapter 7); and the costs and clinical effectiveness of individual care modalities. At the same time a new Commission for Health Improvement will support and oversee the quality of clinical governance and of clinical services.

Early reactions to the new White Paper from health policy pundits were predictable and variable. For Maynard it was 'full of ambiguities and management challenges' and led to 'disorganisation time again' (1998: 20). For others the new start and promise of a 'third way' of running the NHS (i.e. somewhere between centralized command-and-control and the exigencies of the market) was welcome. Ham regarded the White Paper as 'one of the most remarkable documents on the NHS ever published' (Health Service Journal 1997: 11), whilst George feared that 'the proposed changes may just move the same old difficult questions about resources, rationing and the desires of service users and carers from health authorities to a new set of organisations – the primary care groups (George 1998: 20).

Certainly, anyone reading the White Paper of 1997 who is familiar with the historical developments in the NHS which we described in Chapter 7 will be conscious of some underlying continuities, even within an overall message of change. Here we are not referring to those elements of the NHS retained by New Labour from earlier reforms. Rather we are thinking of the continuing pressures to restructure and reorganize; the persistent expression of concerns about local problems and national priorities; and the ever-more differentiated attempts to integrate what clinicians actually do on a day-to-day basis (including the effectiveness of that) with questions of affordability, fairness and equality of access.

Where then do we see the implications for palliative care specifically? An early commentary from Tebbit (1998) saw opportunities and concerns. For example, on the positive side, the continuing emphasis on health needs assessment provides the context for placing palliative care needs within local Health Improvement Programmes, especially with emphasis upon the non-cancer population. This could mean a much more consistent approach than has yet been seen to the question of 'palliative care for all'. At a national level two clear opportunities could be identified for influencing wider questions of clinical care. Here the targets of palliative care professional and representative organizations would be the National Service Frameworks and the National Institute for Clinical Excellence. We would argue that some of the developments reviewed in this book and elsewhere (Robbins 1998) make palliative care reasonably well prepared for this. As we have noted, the palliative care movement has become more sophisticated in recent years in influencing matters of national policy and clearly an evidence-based culture has begun to inform the delivery of palliative care services (Higginson 1997; Robbins 1998).

More negatively, Tebbit (1998) also noted some of the problems for palliative care emanating from the White Paper. Specifically, the task of negotiating with around 100 health commissions would be replaced by the far greater question of collaboration with some 500 primary care groups (in England). Moreover, lying beyond this was the question of how far the primary care groups and their Welsh, Scottish and Northern Irish variants would be constrained by national policy frameworks relating to palliative care – again a deep-seated issue which, as we have seen, has confronted the NHS over several decades.

Writing before the publication of the 1997 NHS White Paper, Bosanquet suggested that the role of specialist palliative care services should change in three key ways. First, there should be an increased emphasis on an educational role; second, there should be greater partnership between specialist palliative care and other service providers, such as nursing homes and primary health care teams; third, there should be more opportunities for 'shared care' (Bosanquet 1997: 1294). In a similar vein, the National Council for Hospice and Specialist Palliative Care Services, in a discussion paper published earlier in the same year as the White Paper, made a number of proposals (NCHSPCS 1997a). Uppermost among these was that non-cancer patients must be offered appropriate palliative care, whether living at home, in institutional care, or in hospital. Such expansion would be achieved in three ways: a growth in palliative care joint appointments which cross health authority, social services and voluntary sector boundaries; a growth in palliative care education as an integral part of clinical education; and the development of new care modalities in which a wide range of needs can be met flexibly and in collaboration between providers of health and social care.

Some idea of how such a 'seamless' service might develop may be gleaned from an examination of recommendations made for the reform of community/institutional care for frail elderly people (Burgner 1996; Johnson and Hoyes 1996; Black and Bowman 1997). Four key reforms are advised:

1 The abolition of the division between residential and nursing homes, and its replacement with a spectrum of homes serving different needs.
2 Withdrawing the registration of homes from local authorities and health authorities and placing it with a National Office for Standards of Care.
3 Development of a comprehensive assessment tool covering health and social needs to ensure appropriate placement of all elderly people.
4 Introduction of specialist nurses to ensure adequate application of the assessment process and supervision of care standards.

As Black and Bowman point out, these reforms of the burgeoning institutional care sector would ensure that the most severely disabled older people and those with 'chronically unstable multiple and complex disease' could receive 'proactive' specialist care and supervision (1997: 442). It is interesting to note that the National Council for Hospice and Specialist Palliative Care Services also makes a particular reference to the care of this client group, recognizing that some hospices may wish to alter their status from providers of specialist palliative care to providers of high-quality nursing or respite care. Under this arrangement: '. . . the quality of care they offer will be second to none, setting standards for many of the nursing homes who aspire to do similar work' (NCHSPCS 1997a: 17).

Another feature of the NHS White Paper of 1997 is the creation of Unified Primary Care Group Budgets which will make available the local population's share of the available resources for hospital and community health services. These will have no upper limit on any part, but will have to be apportioned by some means. In this context Brindle (1998) questions the willingness or ability of GPs to fulfil the role earmarked for them and we must speculate whether palliative care might be neglected in favour of other, more readily identifiable needs. One danger which we can foresee centres around the distinction which has developed between 'specialist' and 'generic' palliative care services. The provision of specialist services of all kinds receives little discussion in the White Paper, though the Calman-Hine model adopted for the integration of cancer services is seen as something which could be transferable to other conditions. As Bunch points out, however, the White Paper says little about the future development of specialist services: 'where', 'by whom' and 'how much'? Thus: 'Given the focus on primary care that is clearly the cornerstone of this nation's health-care philosophy, one can predict challenging times ahead for the specialties' (Bunch 1998: 379).

This may well pose problems for palliative care, which in its specialist development to date has placed greatest emphasis upon the role of in-patient services, and where the role of GPs as a force for change has been remarkably limited.

The 1997 White Paper on the health service therefore poses a range of questions, opportunities and challenges to the hospice and palliative care movement. On the evidence of the 1989 White Paper (Department of Health 1989), our prediction would be that palliative care providers will work with the grain of new developments, achieving further integration with the spectrum of health and social care services. The position of the independent hospices will be particularly interesting in this respect. In recent times the independent hospices have been seeking to clarify their relationship with the wider provision of palliative care. We sense that this is less about isolationism than wishing to retain some control over the independent ethic which first stimulated their development. It seems un-likely however that the growth of specialist in-patient hospices reported in earlier chapters will be sustained in the early decades of the twenty-first century. It may be the case though that some hospices will adopt a less specialist role for themselves, for example in the direction of respite care referred to above (NCHSPCS 1997a). Moving more in the direction of long-term facilities for the population of people with non-malignant life-limiting conditions could be an important role for hospices and one which would gain support in their local communities.

In general however the challenge to the hospice and palliative care move-ment in the UK posed by the 1997 White Paper on the NHS revolves around how far it can build on its existing relationships with primary care to consolidate further its provision of services in the community. In this respect it will be interesting to see what contribution will be made by the newly formed academic departments of palliative care – most of which have a strong bias towards hospital-based services. Overall, the hospice and palliative care movement has proved its adaptability to new waves of change in the NHS. To meet the challenges of the 1997 White Paper we suggest that it must now give further attention to the evidence base for its activity; the primary–secondary care interface; and a new and more proactive partnership with social services.

Unfinished agendas

In these closing paragraphs we will not attempt a summary of the many interlocking issues which will determine the future for palliative care. One such effort as it relates to matters of policy and practice can be found in an occasional paper of the National Council for Hospice and Specialist Palli-ative Care Services, and we would recommend this for its consideration of the 'very probably', the 'probably' and the 'imponderables' (NCHSPCS 1997c: 16–19). Our preference would be to look beyond the sectional interests of the main palliative care stakeholders, to conclude with reference to the wider perspective. Palliative care, it seems to us, is a matter of enormous importance to the twenty-first century and we see that importance in three ways.

At the *individual* level, a growing proportion of the population will end their lives in ways which might benefit from the interventions of palliative care practitioners. As sociologists we are of course nervous about such a categorical statement. We have intimated at various points that the 'holistic', 'reformist' and 'person-centred' claims of palliative care may mask other effects. So it is that the 'discipline' of palliative care is made up of both bodies of knowledge and strategies of power whereby docile bodies, minds and souls may be manipulated, controlled and brought under the gaze of a new governance (Fox 1993). At the same time we would like to think that a 'new reflexivity' within palliative care, of the kind that we called for earlier in this chapter, might set up from within palliative care itself certain strategies of resistance to this process. We also suspect that if more empirical work using sociological and anthropological methods and approaches was conducted in palliative care settings (e.g. Hockey 1990; Lawton 1998) then we would have a greater possibility of picking up individually resistant voices among those who receive palliative care. In this way palliative care could go on with its mission to help a greater number of individuals in need, but do so with greater sensitivity, openness and flexibility. We have no doubt that palliative care at the individual level would be much improved as a result.

At the *social* level, many creative opportunities face palliative care. Above all, we see these in the context of palliative care as a major public issue. To date, palliative care has influenced the public in certain crucial ways. It has gained public support from its work through significant and sustained charitable giving. It has also involved members of the public in voluntary work which is integral to the organization and delivery of its services. Palliative care also, in a modest way, influences public discussions; these however relate chiefly to the question of euthanasia and are almost always oppositional in character. What is lacking is a sustained attention not just to the day-to-day business of providing services (and we do of course understand how easy it may be to become absorbed in these) but to questions of wider public debate. In particular we regard public *education* as a missed opportunity for palliative care (Clark 1997b). As palliative care becomes more specialized there is a great danger that a professional–public gulf could open up and deepen. This would result in a failure to influence and to transform the culture and experience of dying within contemporary culture. Here the problems of alleged 'routinization' and 'medicalization' do become of pressing concern. For as palliative care specialists become caught up and absorbed in such issues, so the wider social mission may be lost. We believe that this is a dilemma both for palliative care managers (preoccupied with standards, budgets, market position and inter-sectoral boundaries) just as it is for clinicians (narrowly focused on symptoms, pharmacological management, and crudely positivistic and reductionist 'evidence'). To both we say: first start to talk again to each other and then refocus on the wider public which you serve. Yours is a unique knowledge base, too valuable to be squandered on inter- and intra-professional jealousies.

Finally, there are challenges at the *societal* level. Here we arrive at questions of social justice and equality. In this context, the claims of palliative care must sit alongside those of many other interest groups, both within health care and beyond. We believe that palliative care fully merits consideration at the societal level. How a society cares for its dying and bereaved is indeed a measure of its compassion and worth. Yet the ability of palliative care to make an influence at this level cannot rest simply on emotive appeals. There is the need to marshall evidence, to lobby, to organize and to influence governments at the highest level. The maturation of the hospice and palliative care movement, especially during the course of the 1990s, has achieved a great deal in this regard. Hospice and palliative care protagonists can now justifiably claim membership of a global constituency and we see signs of their influence being brought to bear in the international arena. Yet around the world, many remain excluded from the physical, social, emotional and spiritual support which palliative care offers. The globalization of palliative care delivery remains a huge matter of unfinished business and, as befits late modern cultures, it should develop in diverse and particularistic ways, always sensitive to local conditions. We are of no doubt however that the establishment of palliative care at the societal and global level is surely something worth working for.

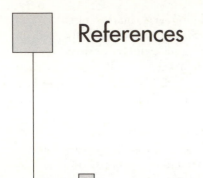

References

Abel, E. (1986) The hospice movement: institutionalising innovation. *International Journal of Health Services*, 16: 71–85.

Abrams, M. (1979) *Beyond Three Score and Ten: A First Report on a Survey of the Elderly*. Mitcham: Age Concern.

Abrams, M. (1980) *Beyond Three Score and Ten: A Second Report on a Survey of the Elderly*. Mitcham: Age Concern.

Addington-Hall, J. and McCarthy, M. (1995) Dying from cancer: results of a national population based investigation. *Palliative Medicine*, 9: 295–305.

Addington-Hall, J.M., MacDonald, L.D., Anderson, H.R., Chamberlain, J., Freeling, P., Bland, J.M. *et al.* (1992) Randomised controlled trial of effects of co-ordinating care for terminally ill cancer patients. *British Medical Journal*, 305: 1317–22.

Ahmedzai, S. (1993) The medicalization of dying: a doctor's view, in D. Clark (ed.) *The Future for Palliative Care*. Buckingham: Open University Press.

Ahmedzai, S. (1994) A defence of medicalization (editorial). *Progress in Palliative Care*, 2: 121–5.

Ahmedzai, S. (1995) Palliative care for all? (editorial). *Progress in Palliative Care*, 3: 77–9.

Ahmedzai, S. (1996) Making a success out of life's failure. *Progress in Palliative Care*, 4: 1–3.

Ahmedzai, S., Morton, A., Reid, J.T. and Stevenson, R.T. (1988) Quality of death from lung cancer: patients' reports and relatives' retrospective opinions, in M. Watson, S. Greer and C. Thomas (eds) *Psychosocial Oncology*. Oxford: Pergamon.

Ahmedzai, S., Mallett, K., Brooks, D. and Johnson, I.S. (1996) 'What are hospices doing now? An update on the survey of clinical practices in UK and Ireland palliative care services'. Paper presented at the Palliative Care Research Forum, Coventry, 6–7 November 1996.

Ahronheim, J.C. (1997) End of life issues for very elderly women: incurable and terminal illness. *Journal of the American Women's Association*, 52: 47–51.

Ahronheim, J.C., Morrison, R.S., Baskin, S.A., Morris, J. and Meier, D.E. (1996) Treatment of the dying in the acute care hospital: advanced dementia and metastatic cancer. *Archives of Internal Medicine*, 156: 2094–100.

Aitken-Swann, J. (1959) Nursing the late cancer patient at home: the family's impressions. *Practitioner*, 183: 64–9.

Andreski, S. (1984) *Max Weber's Insights and Errors*. London: Routledge and Kegan Paul.

Arber, S. and Ginn, J. (1990) The meaning of informal care: gender and the contribution of elderly people. *Ageing and Society*, 10: 429–54.

Arber, S. and Ginn, J. (1992) Class and caring: a forgotten dimension. *Sociology*, 26: 619–34.

Ariès, P. (1976) *Western Attitudes towards Death: from the Middle Ages to the Present*. London: Johns Hopkins University Press.

Ariès, P. (1981) *The Hour of Our Death*. New York: Knopf.

Armstrong, D. (1983) The fabrication of nurse–patient relationships. *Social Science and Medicine*, 17: 457–60.

Armstrong, D. (1984) The patient's view. *Social Science and Medicine*, 18: 737–44.

Armstrong, D. (1987) Silence and truth in death and dying. *Social Science and Medicine*, 24: 651–7.

Armstrong, D. (1995) The rise of surveillance medicine. *Sociology of Health and Illness*, 17: 393–404.

Arney, W.R. and Bergen, B.J. (1984) *Medicine and the Management of the Living*. Chicago: University of Chicago Press.

Asch, David A. (1996) The role of critical care nurses in euthanasia and assisted suicide. *New England Journal of Medicine*, 334: 1374–9.

Audit Commission (1997) *The Coming of Age: Improving Care Services for Older People*. London: Audit Commission.

Bamford, C. (1994) *Grandparents' Lives. Men and Women in Later Life*. Edinburgh: Age Concern Scotland.

Bauman, Z. (1992) *Mortality, Immortality and Other Life Strategies*. Cambridge: Polity Press.

Beck, U. (1992) *Risk Society: Towards a New Modernity*. London: Sage.

Bennett, M. and Corcoran, G. (1994) The impact on community palliative care services of a hospital palliative care team. *Palliative Medicine*, 8: 237–44.

Bennett, M., Alison, D. and Simpson, K. (1994) Care of dying patients in hospital. Palliative care teams have helped (letter). *British Medical Journal*, 309: 1017.

Benoliel-Quint, J.C. (1977) Nurses and the human experience of dying, in H. Feifel (ed.) *New Meanings of Death*. New York, London: Macmillan.

Benzeval, M., Judge, K. and Whitehead, M. (1995) *Tackling Inequalities in Health: An Agenda for Action*. London: King's Fund.

Beresford, L. (1993) *The Hospice Handbook*. Boston: Little, Brown.

Berger, P.L. (1973) *The Social Reality of Religion*. Harmondsworth: Penguin.

Berger, P.L. and Luckmann, T. (1971) *The Social Construction of Reality*. Harmondsworth: Penguin.

Berger, P.L., Berger, B. and Kellner, H. (1973) *The Homeless Mind*. Harmondsworth: Penguin.

Beveridge, W. (1942) *Social Insurance and Allied Services*, Cmnd 6404. London: HMSO.

Biswas, B. (1993) Medicalization: a nurse's view, in D. Clark (ed.) *The Future for Palliative Care*. Buckingham: Open University Press.

Black, D. and Bowman, C. (1997) Community institutional care for frail elderly people. *British Medical Journal*, 315: 441–2.

Bloor, M. (1977) Professional autonomy and client exclusion: a study in ENT clinics, in M. Wadsworth and D. Robinson (eds) *Studies in Everyday Medical Life*. London: Martin Robertson.

Blyth, A.C. (1990) Audit of terminal care in a general practice. *British Medical Journal*, 300: 983–6.

Booth, T. (1985) *Old People's Homes and the Outcome of Care*. Aldershot: Gower.

Bosanquet, N. (1997) New challenge for palliative care. To share its special mission with a wider audience (editorial). *British Medical Journal*, 314: 1294.

Bourdieu, P. (1984) *Distinction: A Social Critique of the Judgement of Taste*. London: Routledge.

Bowlby, J. (1980) *Attachment and Loss, Vol III. Loss, Sadness and Depression*. London: Hogarth Press.

Bowling, A. (1992) Management. Setting priorities in health: the Oregon experiment (Part 2). *Nursing Standard*, 6(38): 28–30.

Boyd, K. (1995a) The development of home care in the UK. *Palliative Care Today*, 4(4): 46–7.

Boyd, K. (1995b) The role of specialist home care teams: views of general practitioners in South London. *Palliative Medicine*, 9: 138–44.

Bradshaw, A. (1996) The spiritual dimension of hospice: the secularisation of an ideal. *Social Science and Medicine*, 43: 409–20.

Bradshaw, J. (1972) A taxonomy of social need, in G. McLachlan (ed.) *Problems and Progress in Medical Care*. Oxford: Oxford University Press.

Brindle, D. (1998) Depth charge. *The Guardian* (Society), 11 March: 19.

Brodsky, M.S. (1995) Testicular cancer survivors' impressions of the impact of the disease on their lives. *Qualitative Health Research*, 5, February: 78–96.

Bruce, S. (1996) *Religion in the Modern World: From Cathedrals to Cults*. Oxford: Oxford University Press.

Bryman, A. (1992) *Charisma and Leadership in Organisations*. London: Sage.

Buckingham, R.W. (1996) *The Handbook of Hospice Care*. New York: Prometheus Books.

Buckland, P. (1997) Hospice in Southern Africa, in C. Saunders and R. Kastenbaum (eds) *Hospice Care on the International Scene*. New York: Springer.

Bunch, C. (1998) Challenging times for specialist services. *British Medical Journal*, 316: 378–81.

Burgner, T. (1996) *The Regulation and Inspection of Social Services*. London: Department of Health.

Bury, M. (1991) The sociology of chronic illness: a review of research and prospects. *Sociology of Health and Illness*, 4, 167–82.

Bury, M. and Holme, A. (1991) *Life after Ninety*. London: Routledge.

Butler, J. (1994) Origins and early development, in R. Robinson and J. Le Grand (eds) *Evaluating the NHS Reforms*. London: King's Fund Institute.

Caddell, D.P. and Newton, R.R. (1995) Euthanasia: American attitudes towards the physician's role. *Social Science and Medicine*, 40: 1671–81.

Cameron, J. and Murray Parkes, C. (1983) Terminal care: evaluation of effects on surviving care before and after bereavement. *Postgraduate Medical Journal*, 59: 73.

Cartwright, A. (1991) Balance of care for the dying between hospitals and the community: perceptions of general practitioners, hospital consultants, community nurses and relatives. *British Journal of General Practice*, 41: 271–4.

Cartwright, A. and Seale, C. (1990) *The Natural History of a Survey: An Account of the Methodological Issues Encountered in a Study of Life before Death*. London: King Edward's Hospital Fund for London.

Cartwright, W. (1996) Killing and letting die: a defensible distinction? *British Medical Bulletin*, 52: 354–61.

Cassell, E.J. (1991) *The Nature of Suffering and the Goals of Medicine*. New York: Oxford University Press.

Challis, L. and Bartlett, H. (1988) *Old and Ill. Private Nursing Homes for Elderly People*. Mitcham: Age Concern England.

Chochinov, H.M., Wilson, K.G., Enns, M., Mowchun, N., Lander, S., Levitt, M. *et al*. (1995) Desire for death in the terminally ill. *American Journal of Psychiatry*, 152: 1185–91.

Christakis, N. (1996) Managing death: the growing acceptance of euthanasia in contemporary society, in R.P. Hamel and E.R. DuBose (eds) *Must we suffer our way to death? Cultural and theological perspectives on death by choice*. [No place of publication]: Southern Methodist University Press.

Cicirelli, V.G. (1997) Elders' end of life decisions: implications for hospice care. *The Hospice Journal*, 12: 57–72.

Clarke, C.L. (1995) Care of elderly people suffering from dementia and their co-resident informal carers, in B. Heyman (ed.) *Researching User Perspectives on Community Health Care*. London: Chapman and Hall.

Clark, D. (1982) *Between Pulpit and Pew: Folk Religion in a North Yorkshire Fishing Village*. Cambridge: Cambridge University Press.

Clark, D. (1991) Contradictions in the development of new hospices: a case study. *Social Science and Medicine*, 33: 995–1004.

Clark, D. (1993a) Death in Staithes, in D. Dickenson and M. Johnson (eds) *Dying, Death and Bereavement*. London: Sage.

Clark, D. (1993b) *Partners in Care? Hospices and Health Authorities*. Aldershot: Avebury.

Clark, D. (1993c) Whither the hospices?, in D. Clark (ed.) *The Future for Palliative Care*. Buckingham: Open University Press.

Clark, D. (1994) At the crossroads: which direction for the hospices? (editorial). *Palliative Medicine*, 8: 1–3.

Clark D. (1997a) Someone to watch over me: Cicely Saunders and St Christopher's Hospice. *Nursing Times*, 26 August: 50–1.

Clark D. (1997b) Public education: a missed opportunity? (invited editorial). *Progress in Palliative Care*, 5: 189–90.

Clark, D. (1998a) Originating a movement: Cicely Saunders and the development of St Christopher's Hospice, 1957–67. *Mortality*, 3: 43–63.

Clark, D. (1998b) An annotated bibliography of the publications of Cicely Saunders: Part 1, 1958–67. *Palliative Medicine* [in press].

Clark, D. (1998c) 'Total pain and disciplinary power in the work of Cicely Saunders,

1957–1967'. Paper presented to the symposium on Pain and Suffering in History, UCLA, Los Angeles, USA, March 1998.

Clark, D. (in preparation) *Cradled to the grave? Care of the dying in the British National Health Service, 1948–67.*

Clark, D. and Haldane, D. (1990) *Wedlocked?* Cambridge: Polity Press.

Clark, D. and Malson, H. (1995) Key issues in palliative care needs assessment. *Progress in Palliative Care*, 3: 53–5.

Clark, D., Neale, B. and Heather, P. (1995) Contracting for palliative care. *Social Science and Medicine*, 80: 1193–201.

Clark, D., Heslop, J., Malson, H. with Craig, B. (1996) '*As Much Help as Possible': Assessing Palliative Care Needs in Southern Derbyshire.* Occasional Paper 19. Sheffield: Trent Palliative Care Centre.

Clark, D., Hockley, J. and Ahmedzai, S. (1997a) *New Themes in Palliative Care.* Buckingham: Open University Press.

Clark, D., Malson, H., Small, N., Mallett, K., Neale, P. and Heather, P. (1997b) Half-full or half-empty? The impact of health reforms on palliative care services in the UK, in D. Clark, J. Hockley and S. Ahmedzai (eds) *New Themes in Palliative Care.* Buckingham: Open University Press.

Clarke, L. (1995) Family care and changing family structure: bad news for the elderly? In I. Allen and E. Perkins (eds) *The Future of Family Care for Older People.* London: HMSO.

Clarke, P. (1996) *Hope and Glory: Britain 1900–1990.* London: Penguin.

Cockburn, M. and Twine, J. (1982) A different kind of day unit. *Nursing Times*, August 18: 1410–11.

Conrad, P. (1975) The discovery of hyperkinesis: notes on the medicalization of deviant behaviour. *Social Problems*, 23: 12–21.

Conrad, P. (1979) Types of medical social control. *Sociology of Health and Illness*, 1: 1–11.

Copp, G. and Dunn, V. (1993) Frequent and difficult problems perceived by nurses caring for the dying in community, hospice and acute care setting. *Palliative Medicine*, 7: 19–25.

Corr, C.A. (1993) Death in modern society, in D. Doyle, G.W.C. Hanks and N. MacDonald (eds) *Oxford Textbook of Palliative Medicine.* Oxford: Oxford University Press.

Corr, C. and Corr, D. (1983) *Hospice Care: Principles and Practice.* New York: Springer.

Cowley, L.T., Young, E. and Raffin, T.A. (1992) Care of the dying: an ethical and historical perspective, *Critical Care Medicine*, 20: 1473–82.

Cowley, S. (1993) Supporting dying people. *Nursing Times*, 89: 52–5.

Crossley, N. (1996) Body-Subject/Body-Power: agency, inscription and control in Foucault and Merleau-Ponty. *Body and Society*, 2: 99–116.

Cumming, E. and Henry, W. (1961) *Growing Old: The Process of Disengagement.* New York: Basic Books.

Dent, O. and Goulston, K. (1982) Community attitudes to cancer. *Journal of Bio-Psychosocial Medicine*, 14: 359–72.

Department of Health (1987) HC(87)4(2). London: Department of Health.

Department of Health (1989) *Working to Patients*, cm 555. London: HMSO.

Department of Health (1990) Press release, 15 March. London: Department of Health.

Department of Health (1994) EL(94)14. *Contracting for Specialist Palliative Care Services*. London: Department of Health.

Department of Health (1995) *NHS Responsibilities for Meeting Continuing Health Care Needs*. London: Department of Health.

Department of Health (1997) *The New NHS: Modern, Dependable*, cm 3708. London: Stationery Office.

Department of Health and Social Security (1981) *Growing Older*, Cmnd 8173. London: HMSO.

Department of Health and Social Security (1983) *NHS Management Enquiry* [The Griffiths Report] DA (83)38. London: DHSS.

Donald, S. and Gordon, D.S. (1991) *Informal Care and Older People: Survey Results from the Aberdeen Informal Support and Care Project*. Edinburgh: Age Concern Scotland.

Donnison, D. and Bryson, C. (1996) Matters of life and death: attitudes to euthanasia, in Social and Community Planning Research, *British Social Attitudes: The 13th Report*. Aldershot: Dartmouth.

Doyle, D. (1992) 'From Assessment to Action'. Address given at the conference 'Palliative Care for All', London, 12 November 1992.

Doyle, D. (1993) Domiciliary palliative care, in D. Doyle, G.W.C. Hanks and N. MacDonald (eds) *Oxford Textbook of Palliative Medicine*. Oxford: Oxford University Press.

Doyle, D. (1994) The future of palliative care, in I.B. Corless, B.B. Germino and M. Pittman, *Dying, Death and Bereavement: Theoretical Perspectives and Other Ways of Knowing*. Boston and London: Jones and Bartlett.

du Boulay, S. (1984) *Cicely Saunders: The Founder of the Modern Hospice Movement*. London: Hodder and Stoughton.

Durkheim, E. (1933) *The Division of Labour in Society*. New York: Macmillan.

Eastaugh, A. (1994) *East Anglian Facilitators' Project in Palliative Care*. London: Cancer Relief Macmillan Fund, Royal College of General Practitioners.

Eastaugh, A. (1996) Approaches to palliative care by primary health care teams: a survey. *Journal of Palliative Care*, 12(4): 47–50.

Elias, N. (1985) *The Loneliness of the Dying*. Oxford: Blackwell.

Ellershaw, J.E., Peat, S.J. and Boys, L.C. (1995) Assessing the effectiveness of a hospital palliative care team. *Palliative Medicine*, 9: 145–52.

Emmanuel, E.J., Fairclough, Diane L., Daniels, Elisabeth R. and Clarridge, Brian R. (1996) Euthanasia and physician-assisted suicide: attitudes and experiences of oncology patients, oncologists, and the public. *Lancet*, 347: 1805–10.

Engebretson, J. (1997) A multiparadigm approach to nursing. *Advances in Nursing Science*, 20: 21–33.

Engel, G. (1961) Is grief a disease? *Psychosomatic Medicine*, 23: 18–22.

Engel, G. (1962) *Psychological Development in Health and Disease*. Philadelphia: Saunders.

Equal Opportunities Commission (1981) *The Experience of Caring for Elderly and Handicapped Dependants: A Survey Report*. Manchester: Equal Opportunities Commission.

Eve, A. and Smith, A.M. (1996) Survey of hospice and palliative care inpatient units in the UK and Ireland 1993. *Palliative Medicine*, 10: 13–21.

Eve, A., Smith, A.M. and Tebbit, P. (1997) Hospice and palliative care services in the UK 1994–5, including a summary of trends 1990–5. *Palliative Medicine*, 11: 31–43.

Expert Advisory Group on Cancer [The Calman-Hine Report] (1995) *A Policy Framework for Commissioning Cancer Services: A Report by the Expert Advisory Group on Cancer to the Chief Medical Officers of England and Wales*. London: Department of Health and Welsh Office.

Exton-Smith, A.N. (1961) Terminal illness in the aged. *Lancet*, 2: 305–8.

Faber-Langendoen, K. (1992) The process of foregoing life sustaining treatment in a university hospital: an empirical study. *Critical Care Medicine*, 20: 570–7.

Faber-Langendoen, K. (1996) A multi-institutional study of care given to patients in hospitals: ethical and practice implications. *Archives Internal Medicine*, 159: 2130–6.

Faulkner, A. and Skilbeck, J. (1995) 'A survey of long-stay attenders in hospice day care'. Poster presentation at Suffering, Coping and Hoping, Second International Conference organized by Trent Palliative Care Centre, 25–27 September 1995. NSPCC Centre, Leicester.

Featherstone, M. (1987) Leisure, symbolic power and the life course, in J. Horne, D. Jary and A. Tomlinson (eds) *Sport, Leisure and Social Relations*. London: Routledge.

Ferguson, C., Nelson, C., Rhodes, P. and Clark, D. (1998) The role of the Macmillan Carer in a new community care service. *International Journal of Palliative Nursing*, 4: 6–13.

Field, D. (1989) *Nursing the Dying*. London: Tavistock/Routledge.

Field, D. (1994) Palliative medicine and the medicalization of death. *European Journal of Cancer Care*, 3: 58–62.

Field, D. (1996) Awareness and modern dying. *Mortality*, 1: 255–66.

Field, D. and James, N. (1993) Where and how people die, in D. Clark (ed.) *The Future for Palliative Care*. Buckingham: Open University Press.

Field, D., Douglas, C., Jagger, C. and David, P. (1995) Terminal illness: views of patients and their lay carers. *Palliative Medicine*, 9: 45–54.

Field, D., Hockey J. and Small N. (1997) *Death, Gender and Ethnicity*. London: Routledge.

Finch, J. (1995) Responsibilities, obligations and commitments, in I. Allen and E. Perkins (eds) *The Future of Family Care for Older People*. London: HMSO.

Finch, J. and Groves, D. (1980) Community care and the family: a case for equal opportunities. *Journal of Social Policy*, 9: 487–511.

Finch, J. and Mason, J. (1990) Filial obligations and support for elderly people. *Ageing and Society*, 10: 151–75.

Finch, J. and Mason, J. (1993) *Negotiating Family Responsibilities*. London: Routledge.

Finch, J. and Summerfield, P. (1991) Social reconstruction and the emergence of companionate marriage, 1945–59, in D. Clark (ed.) *Marriage, Domestic Life and Social Change*. London: Routledge.

Finlay, I.G. and Jones, R.V.H. (1995) Definitions in palliative care. *British Medical Journal*, 311: 754.

Fisher, R.A. and McDaid, P. (1996) *Palliative Day Care*. London: Arnold.

Flynn, R., Pickard, S. and Williams, G. (1995) Contracts and the quasi market in community health services. *Journal of Social Policy*, 24: 529–50.

Foley, K. (1993) Pain assessment and cancer pain syndromes, in D. Doyle, G.W.C. Hanks and N. MacDonald (eds), *Oxford Textbook of Palliative Medicine*. Oxford: Oxford University Press.

Foucault, M. (1973) *The Birth of the Clinic*. London: Tavistock.

Foucault, M. (1977) *Discipline and Punish: The Birth of the Prison*. London: Allen Lane.

Fox, N.J. (1993) *Postmodernism, Sociology and Health*. Buckingham: Open University Press.

Frank, A.W. (1990) Bringing bodies back in: a decade review. *Theory, Culture and Society*, 7: 131–62.

Frank, A.W. (1995) *The Wounded Storyteller*. Chicago: University of Chicago Press.

Frankenberg, R. (1987) Life: cycle, trajectory or pilgrimage? A social production approach to Marxism, metaphor and mortality, in A. Bryman, B. Bytheway, P. Pallatt and T. Keil (eds) *Rethinking the Life Cycle*. London: Macmillan.

Freidson, E. (1970) *Profession of Medicine*. New York: Dodd and Mead.

Freud, S. (1917) Mourning and melancholia, in *The Standard Edition of the Complete Psychological Works of Sigmund Freud*, Vol 14. London: Hogarth Press.

Fulton, G., Madden, C. and Minichiello, V. (1996) The social construction of anticipatory grief. *Social Science and Medicine*, 43: 1349–58.

Garner, J. (1997) Dementia: an intimate death. *British Journal of Medical Psychology*, 70: 177–84.

George, M. (1998) Mixed reception. *Community Care*, 22–28 January: 20–1.

George, R. and Sykes, J. (1997) Beyond cancer?, in D. Clark, J. Hockley and S. Ahmedzai (eds) *New Themes in Palliative Care*. Buckingham: Open University Press.

Gerhardt, U. (1989) *Ideas about Illness: An Intellectual and Political History of Medical Sociology*. Basingstoke: Macmillan.

Giarchi, G.C. (1996) *Caring for Older Europeans: Comparative Studies in 29 Countries*. Aldershot: Arena.

Gibbs, G. (1995) Nurses in private nursing homes: a study of their knowledge and attitudes to pain management in palliative care. *Palliative Medicine*, 9: 245–53.

Giddens, A. (1990) *The Consequences of Modernity*. Cambridge: Polity Press.

Giddens, A. (1991) *Modernity and Self-Identity: Self and Society in the Late Modern Age*. Cambridge: Polity Press.

Giddens, A. (1992) *The Transformation of Intimacy: Love, Sexuality and Eroticism in Modern Societies*. Cambridge: Polity Press.

Glaser, B. and Strauss, A. (1965) *Awareness of Dying*. Chicago: Aldine.

Glennerster, H., Matsaganis, M., Owens, P., with Hancock, S. (1994) *Implementing GP Fund-holding: Wild Card or Winning Hand?* Buckingham: Open University Press.

Glyn Hughes, H.L. (1960) *Peace at the Last*. London: The Calouste Gulbenkian Foundation.

Goffman, E. (1963) *Stigma: Notes on the Management of Spoiled Identity*. Englewood Cliffs, NJ: Prentice Hall.

Goffman, E. (1968) *Asylums: Essays on the Social Situation of Mental Patients and Other Inmates* (originally published 1961). Harmondsworth: Penguin.

Goldin, G. (1981) A protohospice at the turn of the century: St Luke's House, London, from 1893 to 1921. *Journal of the Social History of Medicine and Allied Sciences*, 3: 383–413.

Gomez-Batiste, X., Dulce Fontanals, M., Roca, J., Martinez, F., Valles, E. and Roige-Canals, P. (1997) Rational planning and policy implementation in palliative care, in D. Clark, J. Hockley and S. Ahmedzai, *New Themes in Palliative Care*. Buckingham: Open University Press.

Gorer, G. (1955) The Pornography of Death. *Encounter*, October.

Gorer, G. (1965) *Death, Grief and Mourning in Contemporary Britain*. London: Cressett.

Graham, H. (1983) Caring: a labour of love, in J. Finch and D. Groves (eds) *A Labour of Love: Women, Work and Caring*. London: Routledge.

Green, H. (1988) *Informal Carers*. Series GHS No. 15, Supplement A. London: OPCS.

Griffin, J. (1991) *Dying with Dignity*. London: Office of Health Economics.

Haigh, C. (1990) Adopting the hospice ethic. *Nursing Times*, 86(41): 40–2.

Haines, A. and Booroff, A. (1986) Terminal care at home: perspective from general practice. *British Medical Journal*, 292: 1051–3.

Hammersley, M. (1992) *What's Wrong with Ethnography? Methodological Explorations*. London: Routledge.

Hampe, S.D. (1975) Needs of the grieving spouse in a hospital setting. *Nursing Research*, 24: 113.

Handyside, E. (1995) The needs of people with HIV, their informal carers and service providers, in B. Heyman (ed.) *Researching User Perspectives on Community Health Care*. London: Chapman and Hall.

Harper, R., Ward, A.W., Westlake, L. and Williams, B.T. (1989) *So Birchester Needs a Hospice* . . . Sheffield: University of Sheffield, Department of Community Medicine.

Harris, J. (1996) 'Contract' and 'Citizenship', in D. Marquand and A. Seldon (eds) *The Ideas that Shaped Post-War Britain*. London: Fontana.

Hart, B., Sainsbury, P. and Short, S. (1998) Whose dying? A sociological critique of the 'good death'. *Mortality*, 3: 65–77.

Hastings' Center Report (1995) *Dying Well in the Hospital: The Lessons of SUPPORT*. A special supplement to the Hastings' Center Report, November–December 1995.

Havinghurst, R.J. (1963) Successful dying, in R.H. Williams, C. Tibbits and W. Donaghue (eds) *Processes of Ageing*, Volume 1. New York: Atherton.

Health Committee (1996) *Report on Long-Term Care*. London: HMSO.

Health Services Journal (1997) News focus. 18 December: 10–13.

Henwood, M. (1990) *Community Care and Elderly People*. London: Family Policy Studies Centre.

Hepworth, M. (1984) The mid-life phase, in G. Cohen (ed.) *Social Change and the Life Course*. London: Tavistock.

Higginson, I. (1993) Palliative care: a review of past changes and future trends. *Journal of Public Health Medicine*, 15: 3–8.

Higginson, I. (1995) *Health Care Needs Assessment: Palliative and Terminal Care*. Winchester: Wessex Institute of Public Health Medicine, NHS Management Executive.

Higginson, I. (1997) *Palliative and Terminal Care: Health Care Needs Assessment: The Epidemiologically Based Needs Assessment Reviews.* Oxford: Radcliffe Medical Press.

Higginson, I., Wade, A. and McCarthy, M. (1990) Palliative care: views of patients and their families. *British Medical Journal*, 301: 277–81.

Higginson, I., Priest, P. and McCarthy, M. (1994) Are bereaved family members a valid proxy for a patient's assessment of dying? *Social Science and Medicine*, 3: 553–7.

High, D.M. (1993) Why are elderly people not using advance directives? *Journal of Ageing and Health*, 5: 497–515.

Hillier, K. (1983) Terminal care in the United Kingdom, in C. Corr and D. Corr (eds) *Hospice Care: Principles and Practice.* London: Faber and Faber.

Hinton, J. (1963) The physical and mental distress of the dying. *Quarterly Journal of Medicine*, new series, XXXII, No. 125, January: 1–20.

Hinton, J. (1972) *Dying.* Harmondsworth: Penguin.

Hinton, J. (1979) Comparison of places and policies for terminal care. *Lancet*, 6 January: 29–32.

Hinton, J. (1980) Whom do dying patients tell? *British Medical Journal*, 281: 1328–30.

Hinton, J. (1994) Can home care maintain an acceptable quality of life for patients with terminal cancer and their relatives? *Palliative Medicine*, 8: 183–96.

Hinton, J. (1996) How reliable are relatives' retrospective reports of terminal illness? Patients' and relatives' accounts compared. *Social Science and Medicine*, 43: 1229–36.

Hockey, J. (1988) Residential care and the maintenance of social identity: negotiating the transition to institutional life, in M. Jefferys (ed.) *Growing Old in the Twentieth Century.* London: Routledge.

Hockey, J. (1990) *Experiences of Death: An Anthropological Account.* Edinburgh: Edinburgh University Press.

Hockley, J. (1989) Caring for the dying in acute hospitals. *Nursing Times*, 85 (39 Occasional Paper): 47–50.

Hockley, J. (1996) The development of a palliative care team at the Western General Hospital, Edinburgh. *Supportive Care in Cancer*, 4: 77–81.

Hockley, J. (1997) The evolution of the hospice approach, in D. Clark, J. Hockley and S. Ahmedzai (eds) *New Themes in Palliative Care.* Buckingham: Open University Press.

Hockley, J. and Mowatt, M. (1996) Rehabilitation, in C.A. Fisher and P. McDaid (eds) *Palliative Day Care.* London: Arnold.

Holmes, B. and Johnson, A. (1988) *Cold Comfort. The Scandal of Private Rest Homes.* London: Souvenir Press.

Howarth, G. and Jefferys, M. (1996) Euthanasia: sociological perspectives. *British Medical Bulletin*, 52: 376–85.

Hoyland (1997) Thanks NHS, for a rotten way to die. *Independent* tabloid, 22 April: 8–9.

Hoyt, J.W. (1995) Medical futility, *Critical Care Medicine*, 23: 621–2.

Hunt, M. (1991) The identification and provision of care for the terminally ill at home by 'family' members. *Sociology of Health and Illness*, 13: 375–95.

Hunt, R. (1997) Place of death of cancer patients: choice versus constraint. *Progress in Palliative Care*, 5: 238–41.

Hunt, R., Maddocks, I., Roach, D. and McLeod, A. (1995) The incidence of requests for a quicker terminal course (letter). *Palliative Medicine*, 9: 167–8.

Illich, I. (1976) *Limits to Medicine. Medical Nemesis: The Expropriation of Health*. Harmondsworth: Penguin.

Jackson, A. and Eve, A. (1997) Hospice in Great Britain, in C. Saunders and R. Kastenbaum (eds) *Hospice Care on the International Scene*. New York: Springer.

James, N. (1994) From vision to system: the maturing of the hospice movement, in R. Lee and D. Morgan (eds) *Death Rites: Law and Ethics at the End of Life*. London: Routledge.

James, N. and Field, D. (1992) The routinization of hospice: charisma and bureaucratization. *Social Science and Medicine*, 34: 1363–75.

James, V. (1986) 'Care and work in nursing the dying: a participant study in a continuing care unit', unpublished PhD thesis. Aberdeen University.

James, V. and Field, D. (1996) Who has the power? Some problems and issues affecting the nursing care of dying patients. *European Journal of Cancer Care*, 5: 73–80.

Jefferys, M. (1996) Cultural aspects of ageing: gender and intergenerational issues. *Social Science and Medicine*, 43: 681–7.

Jennings, A.C. and George, R. (1996) Palliative care of HIV diseases and AIDS. *Progress in Palliative Care*, 4: 44–7.

Johnson, I.S., Rogers, C., Biswas, B. and Ahmedzai, S. (1990) What do hospices do? A survey of hospices in the United Kingdom and Republic of Ireland. *British Medical Journal*, 300: 791–3.

Johnson, M. and Hoyes, L. (1996) *Regulating long-term care: proposals for a single registered care home*. A paper for the Joseph Rowntree Foundation. Bristol: School of Policy Studies, University of Bristol.

Jones, R.V.H., Hunsford, J. and Fiske, J. (1993) Death from cancer at home: the carers' perspective. *British Medical Journal*, 306: 249–51.

Joseph, A.E. and Hallman, B.C. (1998) Over the hill and far away: distance as a barrier to the provision of assistance to elderly relatives. *Social Science and Medicine*, 46: 631–9.

Jujawska Tenner, J. (1997) The beginnings of hospice care under communist regime: the Cracow experience, in C. Saunders and R. Kastenbaum (eds) *Hospice Care on the International Scene*. New York: Springer.

Kane, R.L., Wales, J., Bernstein, L., Leibowitz, A. and Kaplon, S. (1984) A randomised controlled trial of hospice care. *Lancet*, I: 890–4.

Kane, R.L., Klein, S.J., Bernstein, L. and Rothenburgh, R. (1986) The role of hospice in reducing the impact of bereavement. *Journal of Chronic Disability*, 39: 735–42.

Kastenbaum, R. (1969) Psychological death, in L. Pearson (ed.) *Dying and Death*. Cleveland: Western Reserve University Press.

Kastenbaum, R. (1991) *Death, Society and Human Experience*. New York: Macmillan.

Kastenbaum, R. (1997) Hospice care in the United States, in C. Saunders and R. Kastenbaum (eds) *Hospice Care on the International Scene*. New York: Springer.

Kearney, M. (1991) Palliative care in Ireland. *Journal of the Irish College of Physicians and Surgeons*, 20: 170.

Kearney, M. (1992) Palliative medicine: just another specialty? *Palliative Medicine*, 6: 39–46.

Keay, T.J., Taler, G.A., Fredman, L. and Levenson, S.A. (1997) Assessing medical care of dying residents in nursing homes. *American Journal of Medical Quality*, 12: 151–6.

Kellehear, A. (1990) *Dying of Cancer. The Final Year of Life*. Reading, Paris, Philadelphia: Harwood Academic.

Kelner, M. (1995) Activists and delegators: elderly patients' preferences about control at the end of life. *Social Science and Medicine*, 41: 537–45.

Kerr, D. (1993) Mother Mary Aikenhead, the Irish Sisters of Charity and Our Lady's Hospice for the Dying. *The American Journal of Hospice and Palliative Care*, May/June, 13–20.

Killbery, E. (1997) What is the relationship between models of palliative care in cancer and models of palliative care in other disease?, in N. Bosanquet, E. Killbery, C. Salisbury, P. Franks, S. Kite, M. Lorentzon *et al.*, *Appropriate and Cost Effective Models of Service Delivery in Palliative Care*. London: Department of Primary Health Care and General Practice, Imperial School of Medicine at St Mary's.

Kite, S. (1997) How can different models of organisation or bed utilisation improve the care of patients dying in hospital?, in N. Bosanquet, E. Killbery, C. Salisbury, P. Franks, S. Kite, M. Lorentzon *et al.*, *Appropriate and Cost Effective Models of Service Delivery in Palliative Care*. London: Department of Primary Health Care and General Practice, Imperial School of Medicine at St Mary's.

Klein, M. (1948) Mourning and its relation to manic depressive states, in *Contributions to Psycho-analysis, 1921–1945*. London: Hogarth Press.

Klein, R. (1983) *The Politics of the National Health Service*. London: Longman.

Kleinman, A. (1988) *The Illness Narratives: Suffering, Healing and the Human Condition*. New York: Basic Books.

Koch, K.A., Rodeffer, H.D. and Wears, R.L. (1994) Changing patterns of terminal care management in an intensive care unit. *Critical Care Medicine*, 22: 233–43.

Komaromy, C. (1995) 'Death and dying in residential nursing homes for older people: examining the case for palliative care'. Paper presented at the Social Context of Death and Dying, 2nd International Conference, University of Sussex, 15–17 September 1995.

Komaromy, C. (1997) 'Relatives' accounts of the deaths of residents in nursing and residential homes'. Paper presented at Symposium on Social Aspects of Death, Dying and Bereavement, Open University, Milton Keynes, 27 November 1997.

Kübler-Ross, E. (1969) *On Death and Dying*. London: Tavistock.

Kübler-Ross, E. (1975) *Death: The Final Stage of Growth*. Englewood-Cliff: Prentice.

Labour Party (1994) *Passing the Buck: Cost-Shunting from the NHS to Local Authorities*. London: Labour Party.

Labour Party (1995) *Reviewing the NHS*. London: Labour Party.

Lasch, C. (1980) *The Culture of Narcissism*. London: Abacus.

Lawton, J. (1998) Contemporary hospice care: the sequestration of the unbounded body and 'dirty dying'. *Sociology of Health and Illness*, 20, 121–43.

Layzell, S. and McCarthy, M. (1993) Specialist or generic community nursing care for IV/AIDS patients? *Journal of Advanced Nursing*, 18: 531–7.

Leach, E. (1967) *A Runaway World? The Reith Lectures*. London: British Broadcasting Corporation.

Levin, P. (1997) *Making Social Policy*. Buckingham: Open University Press.

Levin, E., Sinclair, L. and Gorbach, P. (1989) *Families, Services and Confusion in Old Age*. Aldershot: Avebury.

Levine, D.N., Cleeland, C.S. and Dar, R. (1985) Public attitudes towards cancer pain. *Cancer*, 56: 2237–9.

Lewis, M. (1989) *Tears and Smiles: The Hospice Handbook*. London: Michael O'Mara.

Lewis, J. and Meredith, B. (1989) Contested territory in informal care, in M. Jefferys, *Growing Old in the Twentieth Century*. London: Routledge.

Lindemann, E. (1944) Symptomatology and the management of acute grief. *American Journal of Psychiatry*, 101: 141–8.

Littlewood, J. (1992) *Aspects of Grief: Bereavement in Adult Life*. London: Routledge.

Lo, B. (1995) End of life care after termination of SUPPORT. *Hastings' Center Report (Special Supplement)*, November–December: 56–8.

Lofland, L. (1978) *The Craft of Dying*. Beverley Hills: Sage.

Lofland, L.H. (1985) The social shaping of emotion: the case of grief. *Symbolic Interaction*, 8: 171–90.

Luczak, J. (1997) Palliative care in Eastern Europe, in D. Clark, J. Hockley and S. Ahmedzai, *New Themes in Palliative Care*. Buckingham: Open University Press.

Luddy, M. (1995) *Women and Philanthropy in Nineteenth Century Ireland*. Cambridge: Cambridge University Press.

Lunt, B. (1985) Terminal cancer care services: recent changes in regional inequalities in Great Britain. *Social Science and Medicine*, 20: 753–9.

Lunt, B. and Hillier, R. (1981) Terminal care: present services and future priorities. *British Medical Journal*, 283: 595–8.

Lunt, B. and Yardley, J. (1988) *Home Care Teams and Hospital Support Teams for the Terminally Ill*. Southampton: Cancer Care Research Unit, Royal South Hampshire Hospital.

Lupton, D. (1995) Perspectives on power, communication and the medical encounter: implications for nursing theory and practice. *Nursing Inquiry*, 2: 157–63.

Lupton, D. (1997) Foucault and the medicalisation critique, in A. Petersen and R. Bunton (eds) *Foucault: Health and Medicine*. London: Routledge.

Maccabee, J. (1994) The effect of transfer from a palliative care unit to nursing homes – are patients' and relatives' needs met? *Palliative Medicine*, 8: 211–14.

McCarthy, M., Addington-Hall, J.M. and Altmann, D. (1997) The experience of dying with dementia: a retrospective study. *International Journal of Geriatric Psychiatry*, 12: 404–9.

McGlone, F., Park, A. and Roberts, C. (1996) Relative values: kinship and friendship, in Social and Community Planning Research, *British Social Attitudes: The 13th Report*. Aldershot: Dartmouth.

McIntosh, J. (1977) *Communication and Awareness on a Cancer Ward*. London: Croom Helm.

Mackay, L. (1993) *Conflicts in Care: Medicine and Nursing.* London: Chapman and Hall.

McKeown, T. (1965) *Medicine in Modern Society.* London: George, Allen and Unwin.

McNamara, B. (1997) 'A good enough death?' Paper presented at the Social Context of Death, Dying and Disposal, 3rd International Conference, Cardiff University, April 1997.

McNamara, B., Waddell, C. and Colvin, M. (1994) The institutionalisation of the good death. *Social Science and Medicine,* 39: 1501–8.

McNamara, B., Waddell, C. and Colvin, M. (1995) Threats to the good death: the cultural context of stress and coping among hospice nurses. *Sociology of Health and Illness,* 17: 222–44.

McNulty, E.G. and Holderby, R.A. (1983) *Hospice: A Caring challenge.* Springfield, IL: Charles C. Thomas.

McQuillan, R., Finlay, I., Roberts, D., Brunch, C., Forbes, K. and Spencer, M.G. (1996) The provision of a palliative care service in a teaching hospital and subsequent evaluation of that service. *Palliative Medicine,* 10: 231–9.

Maddocks, I. (1996) Palliative care in the nursing home (editorial). *Progress in Palliative Care,* 4: 77–8.

Manthey, M. (1992) *The Practice of Primary Nursing.* London: King's Fund Centre.

Marie Curie Memorial Foundation (1952) *Report on a National Survey concerning Patients with Cancer Nursed at Home.* London: Marie Curie Memorial Foundation.

Marris, P. (1958) *Widows and their Families.* London: Routledge.

Marshall, Victor W. (1996) Death, bereavement and the social psychology of ageing and dying, in J.D. Morgan (ed.) *Ethical Issues in the Care of the Dying and Bereaved Aged.* Amityville, New York: Baywood.

May, C. (1992a) Individual care? Power and subjectivity in therapeutic relationships. *Sociology* 26: 589–602.

May, C. (1992b) Nursing work, nurses' knowledge and the subjectification of the patient. *Sociology of Health and Illness,* 14: 472–87.

Maynard, A. (1998) Happy days are here again. *Health Service Journal,* 29 January: 20.

Mellor, P. (1993) Death in high modernity: the contemporary presence and absence of death, in D. Clark (ed.) *The Sociology of Death.* Oxford: Blackwell Sociological Review.

Mellor, P.A. and Shilling, C. (1994) Modernity, self-identity and the sequestration of death. *Sociology* 27: 411–32.

Meystre, C.J.N., Burley, N.M.J. and Ahmedzai, S. (1997) What investigations and procedures do patients in hospices want? Interview-based survey of patients and their nurses. *British Medical Journal,* 315: 1202–3.

Mills, C.W. (1967) *The Sociological Imagination.* London: Oxford University Press.

Mills, M., Davies, H.T.O. and Macrae, W.A. (1994) Care of dying patients in hospital. *British Medical Journal,* 309: 583–6.

Mitchell, A. (1997) What investigations and procedures do patients in hospices want? (letter). *British Medical Journal,* 316: 1167.

Mor, V., Greer, D.S. and Kastenbaum, R. (eds) (1988) *The Hospice Experiment.* Baltimore: Johns Hopkins University Press.

Morgan, R. and King, D. (1997) What investigations and procedures do patients in hospices want? (letter). *British Medical Journal*, 316: 1166.

Morris, D. (1997) Palliation: shielding the patient from the assault of symptoms. *Academy Update*, 7(3): 1–11, passim. Gainsville, FL: American Academy of Hospice and Palliative Medicine.

Morris, R.G., Morris, L.W. and Britton, P.G. (1988) Factors affecting the well being of the caregivers of dementia sufferers. *British Journal of Psychiatry*, 153: 147–56.

Mulkay, M. (1993) Social death in Britain, in D. Clark (ed.) *The Sociology of Death*. Oxford: Blackwell/Sociological Review.

Murphy, C. (1989) From Friedenheim to hospice: a century of cancer hospitals, in L. Granshaw and R. Porter (eds) *The Hospital in History*. London: Routledge.

Murray Parkes, C. (1970) Seeking and finding a lost object: evidence from recent studies of reaction to bereavement. *Social Science and Medicine*, 4: 187–201.

Murray Parkes, C. (1979a) Terminal Care: evaluation of in-patient service at St Christopher's Hospice. Part I: Views of surviving spouses on effects of the service on the patient. *Postgraduate Medical Journal*, 55: 517–22.

Murray Parkes, C. (1979b) Terminal Care: evaluation of in-patient service at St Christopher's Hospice. Part II: Self assessments of the effects of the service on surviving spouses. *Postgraduate Medical Journal*, 55: 523–7.

Murray Parkes, C. (1986) *Bereavement: Studies of Grief in Adult Life*. London: Tavistock.

Murray Parkes, C. and Parkes, J. (1984) Hospice versus hospital care – re-evaluation after ten years as seen by surviving spouses. *Postgraduate Medical Journal*, 60: 120–4.

National Health Service Executive (1996) *A Policy Framework for Commissioning Cancer Services: Palliative Care Services*, EL(96)85. Leeds: NHS Executive, 15 October.

NCHSPCS (National Council for Hospice and Specialist Palliative Care Services) (1993) *Needs Assessment for Hospice and Specialist Palliative Care Services: From Philosophy to Contracts*. Occasional Paper No. 4. London: National Council for Hospice and Specialist Palliative Care Services.

NCHSPCS (National Council for Hospice and Specialist Palliative Care Services) (1994) *Palliative Care: Needs, Definitions, Standards: A Consultative Document*. London: National Council for Hospice and Specialist Palliative Care Services.

NCHSPCS (National Council for Hospice and Specialist Palliative Care Services) (1995a) *Information Exchange*, No. 13. London: National Council for Hospice and Specialist Palliative Care Services.

NCHSPCS (National Council for Hospice and Specialist Palliative Care Services) (1995b) *Opening Doors: Improving Access to Hospice and Specialist Palliative Care Services by Members of the Black and Ethnic Minority Communities*. Occasional Paper No. 7. London: National Council for Hospice and Specialist Palliative Care Services.

NCHSPCS (National Council for Hospice and Specialist Palliative Care Services) (1995c) *Specialist Palliative Care: A Statement of Definitions*. London: National Council for Hospice and Specialist Palliative Care Services.

NCHSPCS (National Council for Hospice and Specialist Palliative Care Services) (1995d) *Information Exchange*, No. 14. London: National Council for Hospice and Specialist Palliative Care Services.

NCHSPCS (National Council for Hospice and Specialist Palliative Care Services) (1996a) *Palliative Care in the Hospital Setting*. London: National Council for Hospice and Specialist Palliative Care Services.

NCHSPCS (National Council for Hospice and Specialist Palliative Care Services) (1996b) *Information Exchange*, No. 16. London: National Council for Hospice and Specialist Palliative Care Services.

NCHSPCS (National Council for Hospice and Specialist Palliative Care Services) (1996c) *Information Exchange*, No. 19. London: National Council for Hospice and Specialist Palliative Care Services.

NCHSPCS (National Council for Hospice and Specialist Palliative Care Services) (1997a) *Making Palliative Care Better: Quality Improvement, Multiprofessional Audit and Standards*. London: National Council for Hospice and Specialist Palliative Care Services.

NCHSPCS (National Council for Hospice and Specialist Palliative Care Services) (1997b) *Information Exchange*, No. 21. London: National Council for Hospice and Specialist Palliative Care Services.

NCHSPCS (National Council for Hospice and Specialist Palliative Care Services) (1997c) *Dilemmas and Directions: The Future of Specialist Palliative Care*. Occasional Paper No. 11. London: National Council for Hospice and Specialist Palliative Care Services.

Neale, B. (1991) *Informal Palliative Care: A Review of Research on Needs, Standards and Service Evaluation*. Occasional Paper No. 3. Sheffield: Trent Palliative Care Centre.

Neale, B. (1993) *Informal Palliative Care in Newark: Needs and Services*. Occasional Paper No. 9. Sheffield: Trent Palliative Care Centre.

Neale, B., Clark, D. and Heather, P. (1994) *Palliative Care and the Purchasers: A Study of Recent Developments in Trent Region*. Occasional Paper No. 13. Sheffield: Trent Palliative Care Centre.

Nicholas, A. and Frankenberg, R. (1992) *Towards a Strategy for Palliative Care: A Needs Assessment for Nottingham Health*. Nottingham: Nottingham Health.

Nolan, M., Grant, G. and Keady, J. (1996) *Understanding Family Care*. Buckingham: Open University Press.

O'Brien, T. (1996) Terminal care/palliative care – what do we mean? *Palliative Care Today*, 5(11): 25–6.

O'Donnell, V. (1997) What investigations and procedures do patients in hospices want? (letter). *British Medical Journal*, 316: 1167.

Oliver, G. (1995) Article in *Information Exchange*, No. 15. London: National Council for Hospice and Specialist Palliative Care Services.

O'Neill, P. (1989) Services for the dying. *Nursing Times*, 85(9): 36–7.

O'Neill, W.M., O'Connor, P. and Latimer, E.J. (1992) Hospital palliative care services: three models in three countries. *Journal of Pain and Symptom Management*, 7: 406–13.

OPCS (1992) *General Household Survey: Carers in 1990*. OPCS Monitor SS 92/2. London: OPCS.

Øvretveit, J. (1995) *Purchasing for Health*. Buckingham: Open University Press.

Pappas, D.M. (1996) Recent historical perspectives regarding medical euthanasia and physician assisted suicide. *British Medical Bulletin*, 52: 386–93.

Parker, G. (1990) *With Due Care and Attention: A Review of the Research on Informal Care*. London: Family Policy Studies Centre.

Pattison, E.M. (1978) The living–dying process, in C.A. Garfield (ed.) *Psychosocial Care of the Dying Patient*. New York: McGraw Hill.

Pearson, A. (1988) Primary Nursing, in A. Pearson (ed.) *Primary Nursing: Nursing in the Burford and Oxford Nursing Development Units*. London: Chapman and Hall.

Peräkylä, A. (1989) Appealing to the 'experience' of the patient in the care of the dying. *Sociology of Health and Illness*, 11: 117–34.

Phillips, D.R., Vincent, J. and Blacksell, S. (1988) *Home from Home? Private Residential Care for Elderly People*. Sheffield: University of Sheffield Joint Unit for Social Services Research.

Phillipson, C. (1993) Understanding old age: social and policy issues, in P. Kaim-Caudle, J. Keithley and A. Mullender (eds) *Aspects of Ageing*. London: Whiting and Birch.

Phillipson, C. and Thompson, N. (1996) The social construction of old age: new perspectives on the theory and practice of social work with older people, in R. Bland (ed.) *Developing Services for Older People and their Families*. Research Highlights in Social Work 29. London: Jessica Kingsley.

Pierson, C. (1996) Social policy, in D. Marquand and A. Seldon (eds) *The Ideas that Shaped Post-War Britain*. London: Fontana.

Pijnenborg, L., van der Maas, P.J., Karduan, J.W. *et al.* (1995) Withdrawing or withholding treatment at the end of life: a nationwide study. *Archives of Internal Medicine*, 155: 286–92.

Pincombe, J., O'Brien, B., Cheek, J. and Ballantyne, A. (1996) Critical aspects of nursing in aged and extended care. *Journal of Advanced Nursing*, 23: 672–8.

Pincus, L. (1976) *Death and the Family*. London: Faber.

Pollitt, P.A., Anderson, I. and O'Connor, D.W. (1991) For better or worse: the experience of caring for an elderly dementing spouse. *Ageing and Society*, 11: 443–69.

Porter, R. (1989) The gift relation: philanthropy and provincial hospitals in eighteenth century England, in L. Granshaw and R. Porter (eds) *The Hospital in History*. London: Routledge.

Porter, R. (1996) Hospitals and surgery, in R. Porter (ed.) *The Cambridge Illustrated History of Medicine*. Cambridge: Cambridge University Press.

Prochaska, F.K. (1980) *Women and Philanthropy in Nineteenth Century England*. Oxford: Oxford University Press.

Pugh, E. (1996) An investigation of general practitioner referrals to palliative care services. *Palliative Medicine*, 10: 251–7.

Quint, J.C. (1967) *The Nurse and the Dying Patient*. New York: Macmillan.

Qureshi, H. and Walker, A. (1989) *The Caring Relationship: Elderly People and their Families*. Basingstoke: Macmillan.

Rachels, J. (1975) Active and passive euthanasia. *New England Medical Journal*, 292: 78–80.

Raferty, J.P., Addington-Hall, J.M., MacDonald L.D., Anderson, H.R., Bland, J.M., Chamberlain, J. *et al.* (1996) A randomized controlled trial of the cost effectiveness of a district co-ordinating service for terminally ill cancer patients. *Palliative Medicine*, 10: 151–61.

Randall, F. and Downie, R.C. (1996) *Palliative Care Ethics: A Good Companion*. Oxford, New York: Oxford University Press.

Rando, T.A. (ed.) (1986) *Loss and Anticipatory Grief*. Lexington: Lexington Books.

Ransford, H. and Smith, M. (1991) Grief resolution among the bereaved in hospice and hospital wards. *Social Science and Medicine*, 32: 295–304.

Raphael, B. (1984) *The Anatomy of Bereavement: A Handbook for the Caring Professions*. London: Hutchinson.

Raudonis, B.M. and Acton, G.J. (1997) Theory-based nursing practice. *Journal of Advanced Nursing*, 26: 138–45.

Rees, D. (1997) *Death and Bereavement. The Psychological, Religious and Cultural Interfaces*. London: Whurr Publishers.

Richards, M. (1997) Calman-Hine two years on (editorial). *Palliative Medicine*, 11: 433–4.

Riches, G. and Dawson, P. (1997) 'Shoring up the walls of heartache': parental responses to the death of a child, in D. Field, J. Hockey and N. Small (eds) *Death, Gender and Ethnicity*. London: Routledge.

Robbins, M. (1997) Assessing needs and effectiveness: is palliative care a special case?, in D. Clark, J. Hockley and S. Ahmedzai (eds) *New Themes in Palliative Care*. Buckingham: Open University Press.

Robbins, M. (1998) *Evaluating Palliative Care: Establishing the Evidence Base*. Oxford: Oxford University Press.

Robbins, M., Jackson, P., Brooks, J. and Frankel, S. (1996) Framing the sample in palliative care research: reflections from one district (research abstract). *Palliative Medicine*, 10: 55.

Robinson, L. and Stacy, R. (1994) Palliative care in the community: setting practice guidelines for primary care teams. *British Journal of General Practice*, 44: 461–4.

Robinson, R. (1994) Introduction, in R. Robinson and J. Le Grand (eds) *Evaluating the NHS Reforms*. London: King's Fund Institute.

Rosenmayer, L. and Kockeis, E. (1963) Propositions for a sociological theory of ageing and the family. *International Social Service Journal*, 15: 410–26.

Roy, D.J. quoted in McLennan, M. (1995) Palliative care: an ethical approach, in F. Huser (ed.) *Palliative Care and Euthanasia*. Edinburgh: Campion Press.

Royal College of General Practitioners/Cancer Relief Macmillan Fund (1995) *General Practice Palliative Care Facilitator Project 1992–1994: Report of an Evaluation*. London: RCGP.

Royal College of Nursing (1992) *A Scandal Waiting to Happen?* London: Royal College of Nursing.

Salisbury, C. (1997) What models of palliative care services have been proposed or developed in the UK, Europe, North America and Australia?, in N. Bosanquet, E. Killbery, C. Salisbury, P. Franks, S. Kite, M. Lorentzon *et al.*, *Appropriate and Cost Effective Models of Service Delivery in Palliative Care*. London: Department of Primary Health Care and General Practice, Imperial School of Medicine at St Mary's.

Salvage, A.V., Vetter, N.J. and Jones, D.A. (1989) Attitudes to hospital care among a community sample aged 75 and over. *Age and Ageing*, 17: 270–4.

Salvage, J. (1995) What's happening to nursing: the traditional division of labour between doctors and nurses is changing. *British Medical Journal*, 311: 274–5.

Saunders, C. (1958) Dying of cancer. *St Thomas's Hospital Gazette*, 56(2): 37–47.

Saunders, C. (1961) And from sudden death . . . *Frontier*, Winter: no page numbers.

Saunders, C. (1967) St Christopher's Hospice. *Nursing Times*, 28 July: 988–9.

Saunders, C. (1988) Spiritual pain. *Hospital Chaplain*, March.

Saunders, C. (1993) Foreword, in D. Doyle, G.W.C. Hanks and N. MacDonald, *Oxford Textbook of Palliative Medicine*. Oxford: Oxford University Press.

Saunders, C. (1996) A personal therapeutic journey. *British Medical Journal*, 313: 274–5.

Saunders, C. and Baines, M. (1983) *Living with Dying: The Management of Terminal Disease*. Oxford: Oxford University Press.

Saunders, C. and Kastenbaum, R. (eds) (1997) *Hospice Care on the International Scene*. New York: Springer.

Savage, J. (1995) *Nursing Intimacy: An Ethnographic Approach to Nurse–Patient Interaction*. London: Scutari Press.

Scott, J. (1994) More money for palliative care? The economics of denial. *Journal of Palliative Care*, 16: 35–8.

Scott, S. and Morgan, D. (eds) (1993) *Body Matters*. London: Falmer Press.

Seale, C. (1989) What happens in hospices: a review of research evidence. *Social Science and Medicine*, 28: 551–9.

Seale, C. (1990) Caring for people who die: the experience of family and friends. *Ageing and Society*, 10: 413–28.

Seale, C. (1991a) A comparison of hospice and conventional care. *Social Science and Medicine*, 32: 147–52.

Seale, C. (1991b) Communication and awareness about death. *Social Science and Medicine*, 32: 943–52.

Seale, C. (1991c) Death from cancer and death from other causes: the relevance of the hospice approach. *Palliative Medicine*, 5: 12–19.

Seale, C. (1992) Community nurses and care of the dying. *Social Science and Medicine*, 34: 375–82.

Seale, C. (1995a) Heroic death. *Sociology*, 29: 597–613.

Seale, C. (1995b) Dying alone. *Sociology of Health and Illness*, 17: 377–91.

Seale, C. and Addington-Hall, J. (1994) Euthanasia: why people want to die earlier. *Social Science and Medicine*, 39: 647–54.

Seale, C. and Addington-Hall, J. (1995) Euthanasia: the role of good care. *Social Science and Medicine*, 40: 581–7.

Seale, C., Addington-Hall, J. and McCarthy, M. (1997) Awareness of dying: prevalence, causes and consequences. *Social Science and Medicine*, 45: 477–84.

Seale, C. and Cartwright, A. (1994) *The year before death*. Aldershot: Avebury.

Seale, C. and Kelly, M. (1997) A comparison of hospice and hospital care for people who die: views of the surviving spouse. *Palliative Medicine*, 11: 93–100.

Searle, J.F. (1996) Euthanasia: the intensive care unit. *British Medical Journal*, 52: 289–95.

Sennett, R. (1977) *The Fall of Public Man*. Cambridge: Cambridge University Press.

Seplowin, U.M. and Seravalli, P. (1983) The hospice: its changes through time, in A. Kutscher *et al.* (eds) *Hospice: USA*. New York: Columbia University Press.

Seymour, J.E. (1997) 'Caring for critically ill people: a study of death and dying in intensive care', unpublished PhD thesis. University of Sheffield.

Shanas, E., Townsend, P., Wedderburn, D. *et al.* (1968) *Old People in Three Industrial Societies.* London: Routledge.

Shemmings, Y. (1996) *Death, Dying and Residential Care.* Aldershot: Avebury.

Shilling, C. (1993) *The Body and Social Theory.* London: Sage.

Silverman, D. (1987) *Communication and Medical Practice: Social Relations in the Clinic.* London: Sage.

Simpson, S.H. (1994) A study into the use and effects of do not resuscitate orders in the intensive care units of two teaching hospitals. *Intensive and Critical Care Nursing,* 10: 12–22.

Sims, A., Radford, J., Doran, K. and Page, H. (1997) Social class variation in place of cancer death. *Palliative Medicine,* 11: 369–73.

Sinclair, I. (ed.) (1988) *Residential Care: The Research Reviewed.* London: HMSO/National Institute for Social Work.

Skilbeck, J., Mott, L., Smith, D., Page, H. and Clark, D. (1997) Nursing care for people dying from chronic obstructive airways disease. *International Journal of Palliative Nursing,* 3: 100–6.

Slomka, J. (1992) The negotiation of death: clinical decision making at the end of life. *Social Science and Medicine,* 35: 251–9.

SMAC (Standing Medical Advisory Committee)/SNMAC (Standing Nursing and Midwifery Advisory Committee) (1992) *The Principles and Provision of Palliative Care.* London: HMSO.

Small, N. (1997a) 'Thanatology and the modern hospice movement'. Paper presented at the Social Context of Death, Dying and Disposal, 3rd International Conference, Cardiff University, April 1997.

Small, N. (1997b) Death and difference, in D. Field, J. Hockey and N. Small (eds) *Death, Gender and Ethnicity.* London: Routledge.

Spiller, J.A. and Alexander, D.A. (1993) Domiciliary care: a comparison of the views of terminally ill patients and their family caregivers. *Palliative Medicine,* 7: 109–15.

Stacey, M. (1991) Medical sociology and health policy: an historical overview, in J. Gabe, M. Calnan and M. Bury (eds.) *The Sociology of the Health Service.* London: Routledge.

Stevens, A. and Raftery, J. (1997) Introduction, in I. Higginson, *Palliative and Terminal Care Health Needs Assessment: The Epidemiologically Based Needs Assessment Reviews.* Second Series. Oxford: Radcliffe Medical Press.

Stevens, C.A. and Hassan, R. (1994) Management of death, dying and euthanasia: attitudes and practices of medical practitioners in South Australia. *Journal of Medical Ethics,* 20: 41–6.

Stevenson, M. (1994) Care of dying patients in hospital. Guidelines may have improved care (letter). *British Medical Journal,* 309: 1017.

Stewart, K., Bacon, M. and Bowker, L. (1997) What investigations and procedures do patients in hospices want? (letter). *British Medical Journal,* 316: 1166–7.

Stjernsward, J. (1997) The international hospice movement from the perspective of the World Health Organisation, in C. Saunders and R. Kastenbaum (eds) *Hospice Care on the International Scene.* New York: Springer.

Stone, P.O., Phillips, C., Nabbot, A. and Langstone, P. (1994) Care of dying patients in hospital. Things have improved (letter). *British Medical Journal*, 309: 1017.

Strauss, A.L., Fagerhaugh, S., Suczek, B. and Wiener, C. (1985) *The Social Organization of Medical Work*. Chicago, London: University of Chicago Press.

Stroebe, M. (1996) 'New directions in bereavement research: exploration of gender differences'. Paper presented at the Bereavement Research Forum, Annual Palliative Care Congress, Coventry, UK, November 5–8 1996.

Stroebe, W. and Stroebe, M. (1987) *Bereavement and Health*. Cambridge: Cambridge University Press.

Strong, P. (1979) *The Ceremonial Order of the Clinic: Parents, Doctors and Medical Bureaucracies*. London: Routledge and Kegan Paul.

Strong, P. and Robinson, J. (1990) *The NHS – Under New Management*. Buckingham: Open University Press.

Sudnow, D. (1967) *Passing On: The Social Organization of Dying*. Englewood Cliffs, New Jersey: Prentice Hall.

SUPPORT Project Principal Investigators (1995) A controlled trial to improve care of seriously ill hospitalized patients: the study to understand prognoses and preferences for outcomes and risks of treatment (SUPPORT). *Journal of the American Medical Association*, 174: 1591–8.

Sykes, N.P., Pearson, S. and Chell, S. (1992) Quality care for the terminally ill: the carer's perspective. *Palliative Medicine*, 6: 227–36.

Szasz, T. (1964) *The Myth of Mental Illness: Foundations of a Theory of Personal Conduct*. New York: Harper and Row.

Taylor, H. and Ford, G. (1983) Inequality in old age: an examination of age, sex, and class differences in a sample of community elderly. *Ageing and Society*, 3: 183–208.

Tebbit, P. (1998) Opportunity or threat? *Information Exchange*, 24: 10.

Thompson, P., Itzin, C. and Aberndstern, M. (1991) *I Don't Feel Old. The Experience of Later Life*. Oxford: Oxford University Press.

Thorpe, G. (1993) Enabling more dying people to remain at home. *British Medical Journal*, 307: 915–18.

Timmins, N. (1996) *The Five Giants: A Biography of the Welfare State*. London: Fontana.

Titmuss, R. (1958) *Essays on 'the Welfare State'*. London: Unwin.

Townsend, J., Frank, A.O., Fermont, D., Dyer, S., Karan, O. and Walgrove, A. (1990) Terminal cancer care and patients' preference for place of death: a prospective study. *British Medical Journal*, 301: 415–27.

Townsend, P. (1957) *The Family Life of Old People: An Inquiry in East London*. London: Routledge.

Townsend, P. (1964) *The Last Refuge: A Survey of Residential Institutions and Homes for the Aged in England and Wales*. London: Routledge and Kegan Paul.

Townsend, P. (1981) The structured dependency of the elderly: the creation of social policy in the twentieth century. *Ageing and Society*, 1: 5–28.

Turner, B.S. (1984) *The Body and Society*. Oxford: Blackwell.

Turner, B.S. (1987) *Medical Power and Social Knowledge*. London: Sage.

Turner, B.S. (1992) *Regulating Bodies*. London: Routledge.

Turner, B.S. (1996) *Medical Power and Social Knowledge*, 2nd edition. London: Sage.

Turner, V. (1969) *The Ritual Process*. Chicago: Aldine.

Twigg, J. and Atkin, K. (1994) *Carers Perceived*. Buckingham: Open University Press.

Twigg, J., Atkin, K. and Perring, C. (1990) *Carers and Services: A Review of Research*. London: HMSO/ York: Social Policy Research Unit.

Twycross, R.G. and Lack, S.A. (1983) *Symptom Control in Far-advanced Cancer: Pain Relief*. London: Pitman.

van der Maas, P.J., van Deldon, J.J.M., Pijnenborg, L. and Looman, C.W.N. (1991) Euthanasia and other medical decisions concerning the end of life. *Lancet*, 338: 669–74.

van Gennep, A. (1960) *The Rites of Passage*. London: Routledge and Kegan Paul.

Walby, S. and Greenwell, J. (1994) *Medicine and nursing: professions in a changing health service*. London, Thousand Oaks, New Delhi: Sage.

Walker, A. (1986) Pensions and the production of poverty in old age, in C. Phillipson and A. Walker (eds) *Ageing and Social Policy*. London: Gower.

Walker, A. (1993) Old people in Europe: perceptions and realities, in P. Kaim-Caudle, J. Keithley and A. Mullender (eds) *Aspects of Ageing: A Celebration of the European Year of Older People and Solidarity between Generations*. London: Whiting and Birch.

Walter, T. (1993) Sociologists never die: British sociology and death, in D. Clark (ed.) *The Sociology of Death*. Oxford: Blackwell/Sociological Review.

Walter, T. (1994) *The Revival of Death*. London: Routledge.

Walter, T. (1996) A new model of grief: bereavement and biography. *Mortality*, 1: 7–25.

Walter, T. (1997a) The ideology and organization of spiritual care: three approaches. *Palliative Medicine*, 11: 21–30.

Walter, T. (1997b) *The Eclipse of Eternity: A Sociology of the Afterlife*. Basingstoke: Macmillan.

Ward, A.W.M. (1987) Home care services – an alternative to hospices? *Community Medicine*, 9: 47–54.

Ward, B.J. and Tate, P.A. (1994) Attitudes among NHS doctors to requests for euthanasia. *British Medical Journal*, 308: 1332–4.

Warnes, A.M. (1996) The demography of old age: panic versus reality, in R. Bland (ed.) *Developing Services for Older People and their Families*. Research Highlights in Social Work No. 29. London: Jessica Kingsley.

Webster, C. (1996) *The Health Services Since the War, Vol II: Government and Health Care, the National Health Service 1958–1979*. London: Stationery Office.

Wendell-Moller, D. (1996) *Confronting Death: Values, Institutions and Human Mortality*. New York, Oxford: Oxford University Press.

Wenger, G.C. (1984) *The Supportive Network*. London: Allen and Unwin.

Wenger, G.C. (1989) Support networks in old age: constructing a typology, in M. Jefferys (ed.) *Growing Old in the Twentieth Century*. London: Routledge.

West, P. (1984) The family, the welfare state and community care: political rhetoric and public attitudes. *Journal of Social Policy*, 13: 417–46.

WHO (World Health Organisation) Expert Committee (1990) *Cancer pain relief and palliative care*. Technical Report Series No. 804. Geneva: World Health Organisation.

Whynes, D. (1997) Costs of palliative care, in D. Clark, J. Hockley and S. Ahmedzai (eds) *New Themes in Palliative Care*. Buckingham: Open University Press.

Wilkes, E. (1965) Terminal cancer at home. *Lancet*, April 10: 799–800.

Wilkes, E. (1981) General practitioner in a hospice. *British Medical Journal*, 282: 1591.

Wilkes, E. (1984) Dying now. *Lancet*, April 28: 950–2.

Williams, R. (1989) Awareness and control of dying: some paradoxical trends in public opinion. *Sociology of Health and Illness*, 11: 201–12.

Williams, R. (1990) *The Protestant Legacy: Attitudes to Death and Illness among Older Aberdonians*. Oxford: Clarendon Press.

Williams, R. (1992) Social movements and disordered bodies: the reform of birth, sex, drink, and death in Britain since 1850, in R. Williams (ed.) *Social Research and Social Reform: Essays in Honour of A.H. Halsey*. Oxford: Oxford University Press.

Willmott, P. and Young, M. (1962) *Family and Kinship in East London*. London: Penguin.

Worden, W. (1982) *Grief Counselling and Grief Therapy*. New York: Springer.

Working Group on Terminal Care [The Wilkes Report] (1980) *Report of the Working Group on Terminal Care*. London: DHSS.

Wouters, C. (1990) Changing regimes of power and emotions at the end of life: the Netherlands 1930–1990. *Netherlands Journal of Sociology*, 26: 151–67.

Wright, S. (1990) *My patient – my nurse: the practice of primary nursing*. London: Scutari Press.

Young, M. and Willmott, P. (1957) *Family and Kinship in East London*. Harmondsworth: Penguin.

Zola, I. (1972) Medicine as an institution of social control. *Sociological Review*, 20: 487–503.

Zola, I. (1975) In the name of health and illness: on some socio-political consequences of medical influence. *Social Science and Medicine*, 9: 83–7.

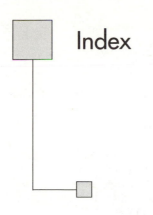

Index

advance directives, 56
  see also euthanasia
ageing, 25–32
  see also older people
AIDS/HIV, 82, 155, 162, 165
Alzheimer's Disease, 18–19
  see also dementia
awareness, 115–18

bereavement, 40–5
  bereavement care, 43
  and ethnicity, 45
body, 15–17, 18
bureaucracy, 105, 118–24

Calman-Hine reforms, 148
Calman-Hine report, 148
cancer, 83, 94–5, 152, 155
cancer charities, *see* Macmillan Cancer
  Relief; Marie Curie Foundation
cardio-pulmonary resuscitation, 100–3
carers, informal, 160–2, 164, 168
charisma, 105
chronic obstructive airways disease,
  158–9, 162
clinical gaze, 66
community care, 26, 34
community care reforms, 140
community nurses, 159–61
  see also district nurses

community nursing services, 159–61
day care, 164–5
home care, 157–65
  see also death, home deaths
practice nurses, 159–61
primary health care teams, 159–61
  see also general practitioners
  see also Macmillan nurses, Marie
  Curie nurses

death
  age at, 30–1
  denial of, 115
  'good' death concept, 27, 63, 79,
    88–94
  'good enough' death concept,
    93–4
  home deaths, 22, 157–9
  late modernity and, 10–12, 21–3,
    56, 176–8
  medicalized death, 115–18
  sequestration and, 15, 31
  social death, 115
  sociology and, 8–10, 11
definitions of palliative care, 80–7
  see also palliative care
dementia, 100, 169
disciplinary power, 116
district nurses, 159–61
  see also community nurses

elderly people, *see* older people
embodiment, 15–17, 178
ethnicity, 44–5
euthanasia
  attitudes to, 49–51
  definitions of, 48
  ethical judgements in, 56–7
  evidence base and, 54–5
  factors affecting request for, 23
  and 'good death', 93
  hospice care and, 54–6
  physician assisted suicide, 50
  professionals' experience of, 53–4
  public opinion on, 50–1, 56–7
  relationship to affluence and
    development, 53
  responding to requests for, 52–7

general practitioners, 159–61, 163
  see also community care
grief, 21, 41–6, 92, 118, 169

holism, 96, 110, 112–13, 156
hospices
  admission criteria, 166
  day hospices, 164–5
  funding, 138–9, 141–2, 149
  future, 94–6
  global development of, 76–8
  health care reforms and, 137,
    139–46
  history and development, UK and
    Ireland, 133–40
  National Health Service and,
    133–40
  philosophy of, 66, 69, 94
  as a reformist movement, 73–8
  St Christopher's Hospice, 72–3, 74,
    92, 119, 134, 135, 166
  US National Hospice Study, 77
hospitals, 99–103, 152–7
  historical development of, 65–7
  hospital palliative care teams, 152–6

iatrogenesis, 116
identity, 15–17
informal care, 32–40, 95
  see also carers, informal

institutional homes, 168–72
intensive care, 51, 123

lived experience, 115

Macmillan Cancer Relief, 106, 152, 163
Macmillan Carer Schemes, 163
Macmillan nurses, 162–3
Marie Curie Foundation, 106
Marie Curie homes, 165
Marie Curie nurses, 162–3
meaning of illness, *see* lived experience
medicalization and medical model,
    113–24, 115–18
  see also death, medicalized death

narratives of illness, suffering, 18–19
National Council for Hospice and
    Specialist Palliative Care Services,
    84, 86, 145, 147, 149, 152, 153,
    154, 180, 185–6
National Health Service (NHS)
  budget allocation, 138–9
  Conservative reforms, impact of,
    139–46
  contracts, 149
  contract monitoring, 142
  general practice fundholding, 146–7
  hospices and, 75, 133–6, 137–8
  internal market in, 140–1, 181
  primary care, 181–2, 184–5
  purchasing cycle, 140–1
  White Paper of 1997, 181–5
need
  assessment of, 144–6
  definitions, 143–4
  health needs assessment models
    applied to palliative care, 143–5
non-cancer disease, 158–9
nursing, 92, 107–9, 111–13
  see also community care
nursing homes, *see* institutional homes

older people, 168–72

pain
  management of, 23
  psychosocial and spiritual aspects,
    see spiritual issues

'total pain', 92, 110
    see also spiritual issues; suffering
see also suffering; symptom
    management
palliative care, 79–103
    approach, 79, 83, 86
    definitions, 80–8
    generic health care services and,
        151–72
    history of, 73–8, 95–102
    medicine, 79, 92, 121
    philosophy, 86
    principles, 87, 104
    and range of services, 95, 151–72
    specialist palliative care, 79, 83, 86
political economy perspective, 116
professionalization, 111
psychiatry, 114
psychological issues
    see also bereavement; spiritual
        issues; suffering

quality of life, 85

religious values, 107–8, 109
research
    ethnography, 166
    randomized controlled trials, 84, 120
routinization, 104–13

Saunders, Cicely, 62, 65, 71–3, 108,
    109, 110, 111
secularization, 107–8, 109
Sheffield 'model', 85
SMAC/SNMAC report, 141
specialist palliative care, 79, 83, 87
spiritual issues, 109–12
    see also suffering; pain, 'total pain'
social death, 12, 26
suffering, 17–21, 23, 51, 54, 66, 68,
    77, 83, 99, 104, 111, 114, 118,
    177
    see also euthanasia
stigma, 114
Sue Ryder homes, 165
SUPPORT study, 101–3
symptom management, 152–7, 163

teamwork, 83
technology, 93, 122
terminal care, 79, 83, 84, 85, 105
    see also euthanasia; symptom
        management

United States of America (USA), 100,
    105

World Health Organization, 83, 85
Wilkes report, 137, 141

THE FUTURE FOR PALLIATIVE CARE
ISSUES OF POLICY AND PRACTICE

David Clark (ed.)

In recent years the independent hospice movement has done a great deal to promote care standards. But many issues remain unsolved. Can and should the hospice approach be translated into other settings? How can care be improved in hospitals, in the community, and in residential and nursing homes? How can such care be costed and evaluated? What new service initiatives are required and how are these affected by changes in government policy? How do planners and practitioners address the ethical and cultural needs of a changing society?

Drawing on a variety of disciplines and specialties in medicine, nursing and the social sciences, expert contributors explore the future for palliative care, paying particular attention to the relationship between policy and practice.

This challenging volume breaks new ground in our thinking about how dying people should be cared for and will be essential reading for practitioners, students and researchers in palliative care.

> This book is timely, engaging, and to the point and crystallises many of the relevant arguments. It deserves to be widely read both within and without palliative care circles.
>
> (*British Medical Journal*)

> This lively book will be of particular interest to those working in palliative care; its treatment of general themes should widen its appeal.
>
> (*Nursing Times*)

> This modestly priced, well-presented book is a useful contribution to palliative care literature.
>
> (*Progress in Palliative Care*)

Contents
Introduction – Where and how people die – Quality, costs and contracts of care – Information care and community care – Developments in bereavement services – HIV/AIDS: lessons for policy and practice – Cultural issues in terminal care – Euthanasia – The medicalization of dying – A doctor's view – Issues in pain management – Whither the hospices? – Index.

Contributors
Sam Ahmedzai, Richard Atkinson, Bronwen Biswas, David Clark, Tony Crowther, Graham Davies, Ann Faulkner, David Field, Shirley Firth, Barry Hancock, Irene Higginson, Nicky James, Brenda Neale, Neil Small, Eric Wilkes.

192pp   0 335 15764 5 (Paperback)